The Funny Side Collection

The Fart Side

Life is a Gas!

(Pocket Rocket Edition!)

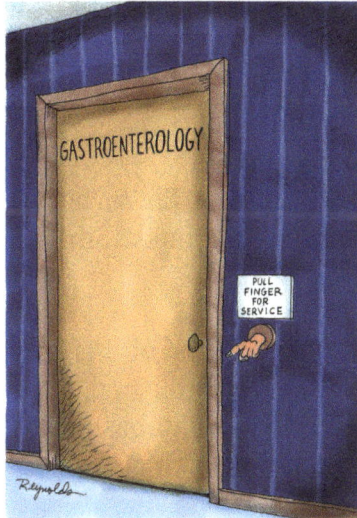

Dan Reynolds

Joseph Weiss, MD

ISBN-13: 978-1-943760-48-0 (Color Pocket Rocket)
ISBN-13: 978-1-943760-49-7 (e-Book Pocket Rocket)
ISBN-13: 978-1-943760-56-5 (Color Print Expanded)
ISBN-13: 978-1-943760-61-9 (e-Book Expanded)

The Fart Side: Life is a Gas!

Because of Bob's excessive gas, the Alaskan natural gas pipeline makes a detour...

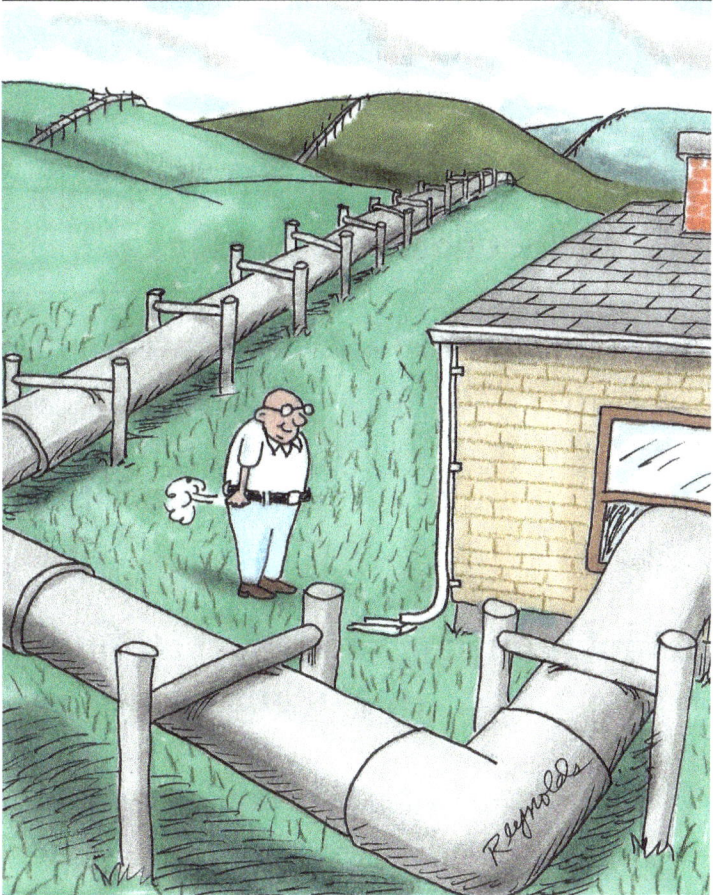

The clear majority of the gasses in intestinal farts, with nitrogen, hydrogen, carbon dioxide, methane, and oxygen contributing 99.9% by volume are odorless

The minor 0.1% of intestinal gasses that are not odorless includes indoles, skatoles, thiols, sulfhydryls, mercaptans, and aromatic fatty acids.

A surprising percentage of the normal population (predominantly males) profess enjoyment and pleasure with the olfactory stimulation generated by their own farts, but not those of others.

The aroma of a fart can be an indicator of intestinal health.

The Fart Side: Life is a Gas!

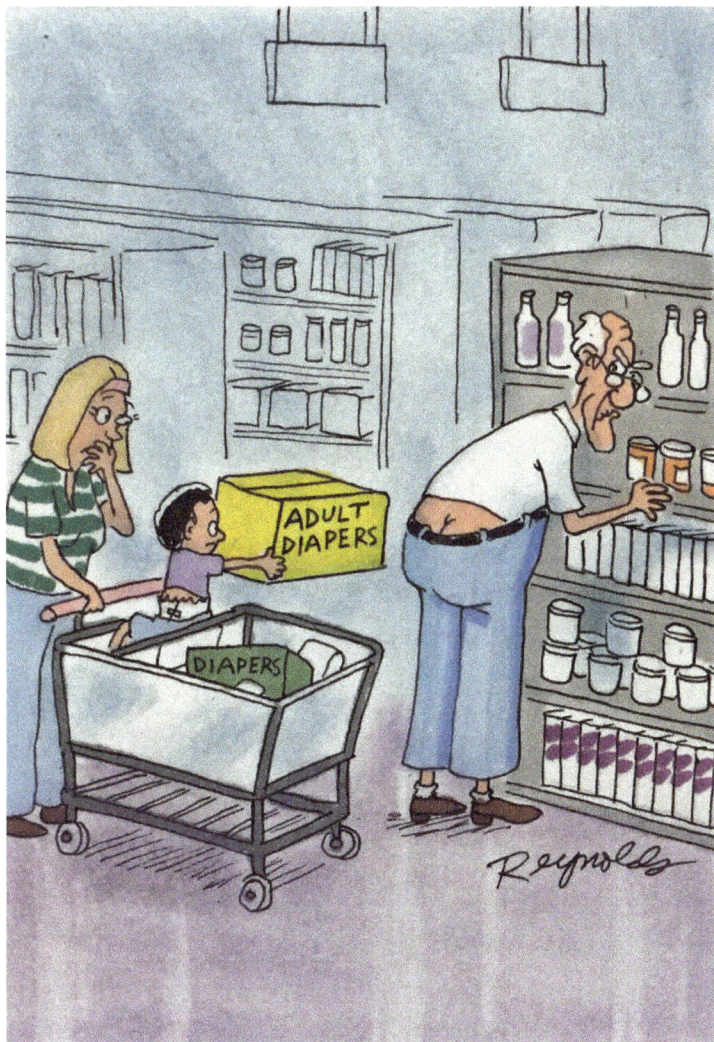

The Funny Side Collection

Indole is used as a constituent fragrance in many perfumes.

The name indole is a portmanteau created from the words indigo and oleum.

Indole was first isolated by the dye industry in treatment of the deep blue indigo dye with oleum.

Indole is widely distributed in the natural environment and can be produced by a variety of bacteria as a degradation product of the amino acid tryptophan.

Skatole (from the Greek το σχατος = feces), or methylindole, is a mildly toxic organic compound belonging to the indole family.

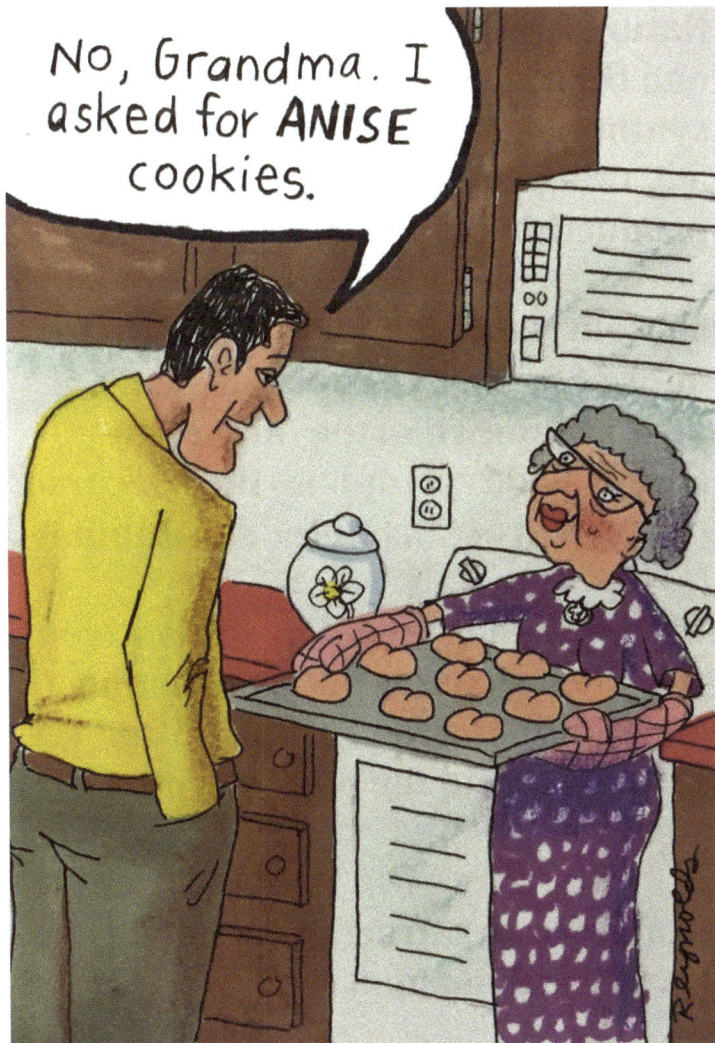

Nature harvested jasmine costs over one thousand times as much as synthetic jasmine, which takes advantage of the commercial production of indole.

Skatole is the primary source of the odor of feces, and is produced from the breakdown of the important amino acid tryptophan, the precursor of the neurotransmitter serotonin.

Tryptophan is an indole derivative and the precursor of the hormone melatonin, the neurotransmitter serotonin, and the plant hormone auxin.

Skatole is an attractant to gravid (pregnant) mosquitos.

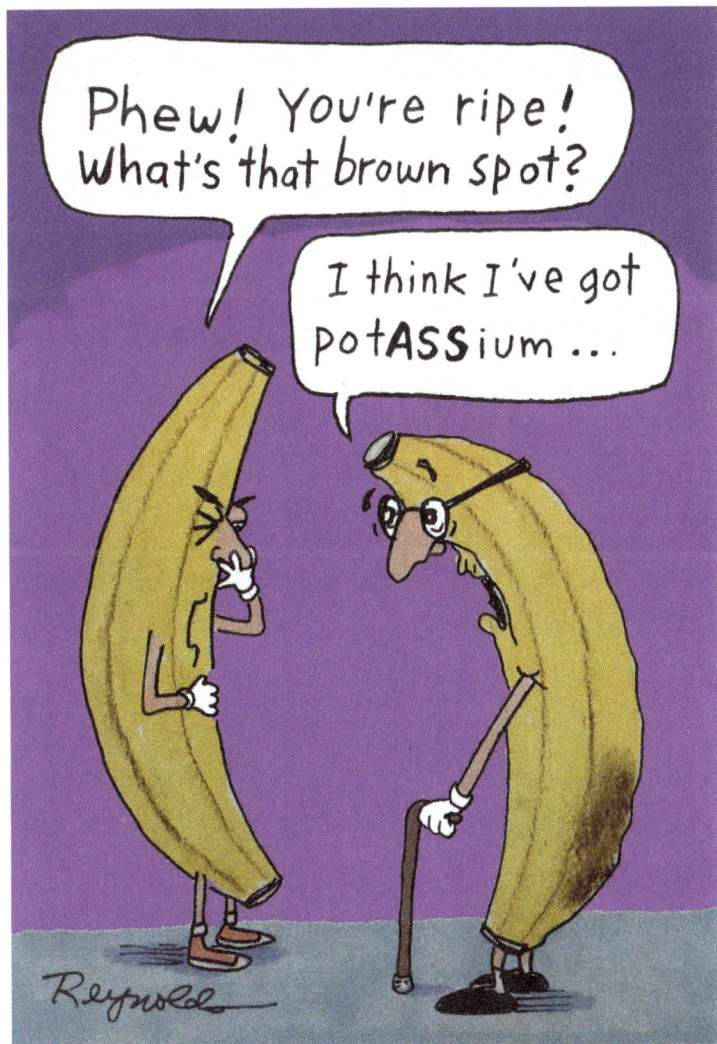

Hydrogen sulfide is known for its characteristic odor of smelling like rotten eggs. Surprisingly women tend to produce more hydrogen sulfide then men.

The small bowel is more than three times as long as the large bowel.

Diet plays a role in hydrogen sulfide production, and cruciferous vegetables such as broccoli, cabbage, cauliflower, and Brussels sprouts are common offenders.

Red meat, beer, garlic, and aromatic spices are other significant contributors to hydrogen sulfide production which contributes to offensive and odiferous intestinal gas.

The Fart Side: Life is a Gas!

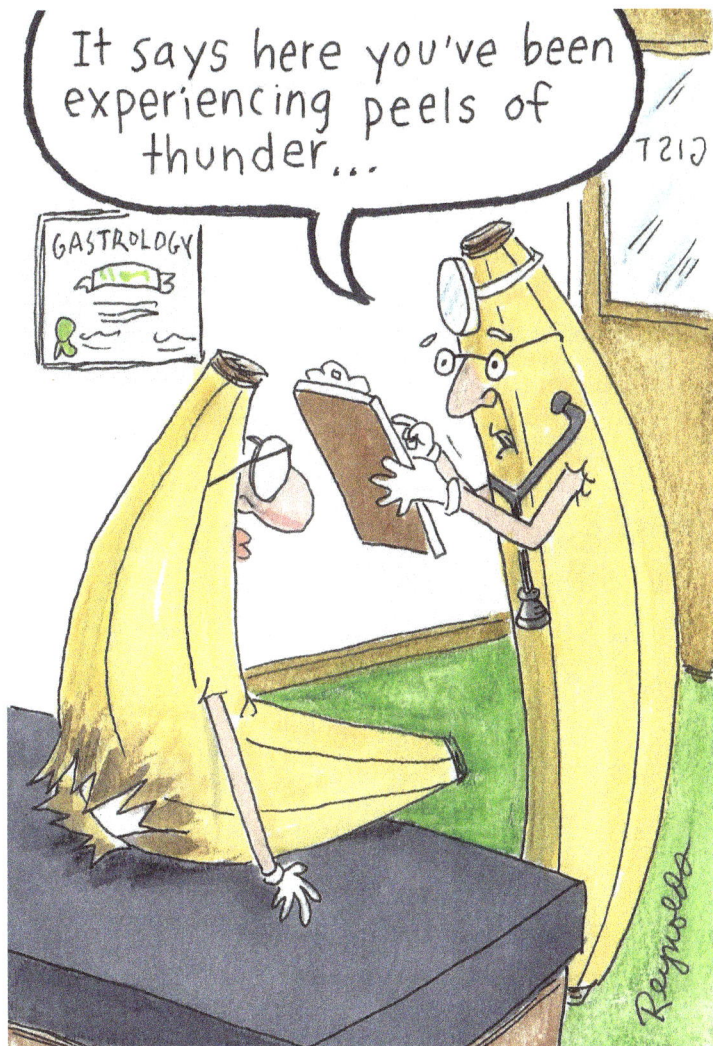

Dried fruits such as apricots are often treated with sulfur products that create odiferous intestinal gasses.

The offensive smell of sulfur products led to several religions ascribing an association between the devil and sulfur.

Activated carbon is used to treat oral poisonings by binding to and preventing the poison from being absorbed by the gastrointestinal tract.

Charcoal biscuits were marketed in the early 19th century as an antidote to flatulence, and are still marketed today for diarrhea, indigestion, flatulence, and as a pet care product.

The Fart Side: Life is a Gas!

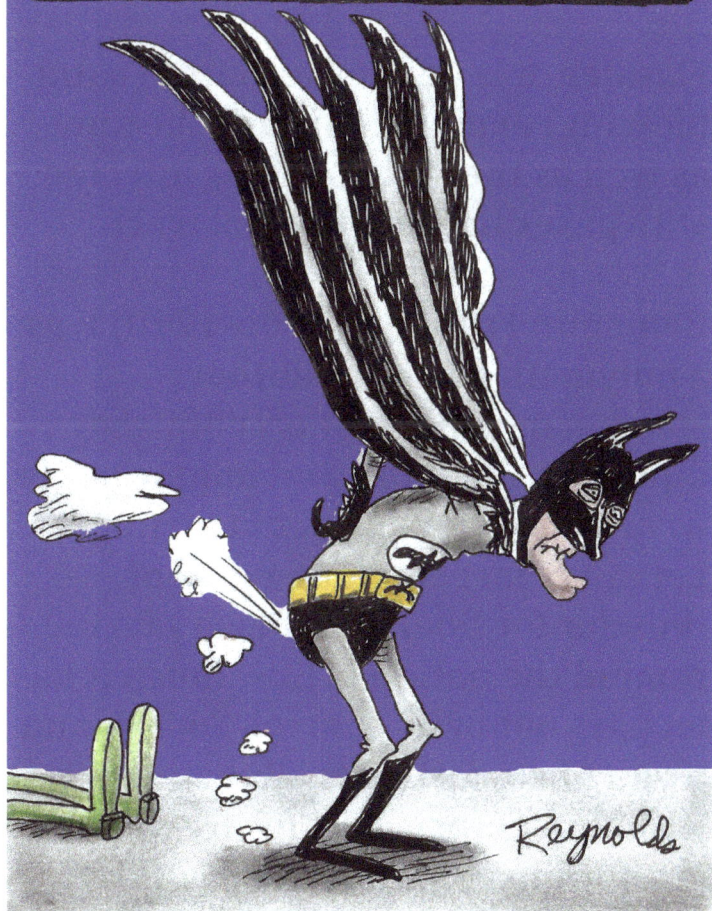

Later in life. Batman would fend off villains with Bat Gas.

The scientific study of flatulence and farting is termed flatology.

Flatulence is defined as flatus (Latin blowing) expelled through the anus, as well as the state of being affected with gases in the intestinal tract.

**Benjamin Franklin (1706-1790) was a polymath scientist, author, statesman, philosopher, publisher, diplomat, inventor, and humorist. He wrote the following about farting:"
Let every fart count as a peal of thunder for liberty. Let every fart remind the nation of how much it has let pass out of its control. So fart, and if you must, fart often. But always fart without apology. Fart for freedom, fart for liberty... and fart proudly!"**

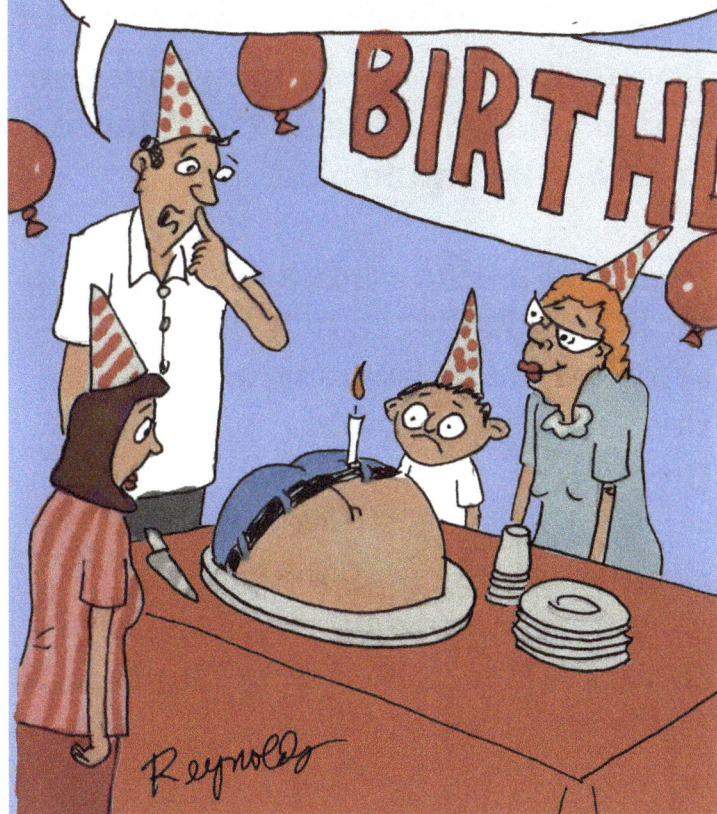

Higher methane concentrations in intestinal gas have been associated with decreased gastrointestinal tract motility and constipation.

Tryptophan is one of the twenty-two amino acids, and is also considered an essential amino acid.

Essential amino acids are those amino acids that cannot be synthesized by humans, and therefore must be obtained through the diet.

Because of its importance as an essential amino acid, tryptophan is a common constituent of most protein foods and supplements.

The Fart Side: Life is a Gas!

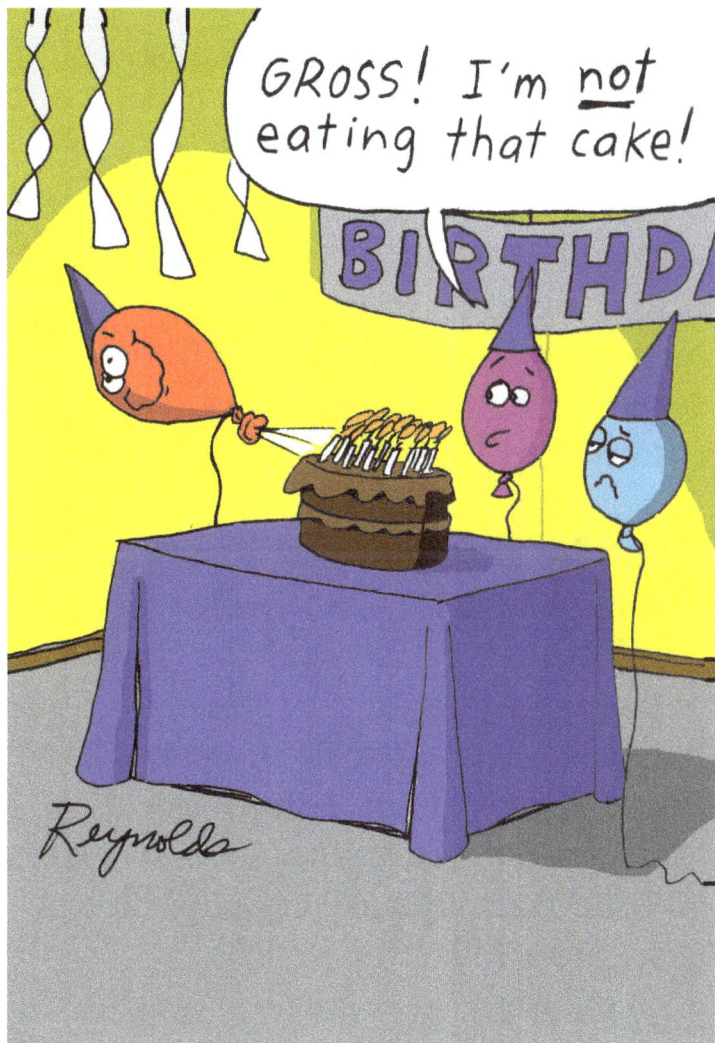

In addition to being heard and smelled, a fart can be seen if the circumstances are right. In the polar zones, at very high altitude, in frigid weather, or even in a walk-in freezer, dropping a fart from exposed buttocks would look much like the steamy cloud of warm breath on a cold winter day.

Frostbite is a real risk for mountain climbers, and for the adventurous climbing Mount Everest the comforts of base camp at an altitude of 17,590 feet may be the last chance they have for a protected bowel movement. At higher altitudes, there are no shelters so their buttocks are exposed to the extreme winds and weather approaching the summit. Frostbutt?

The Fart Side: Life is a Gas!

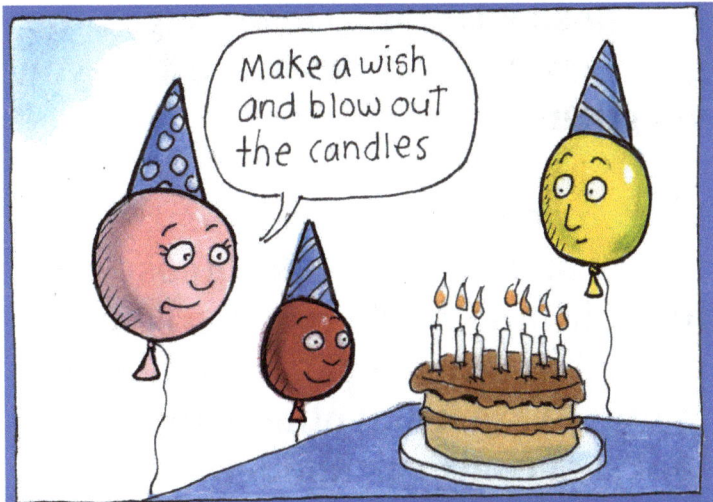

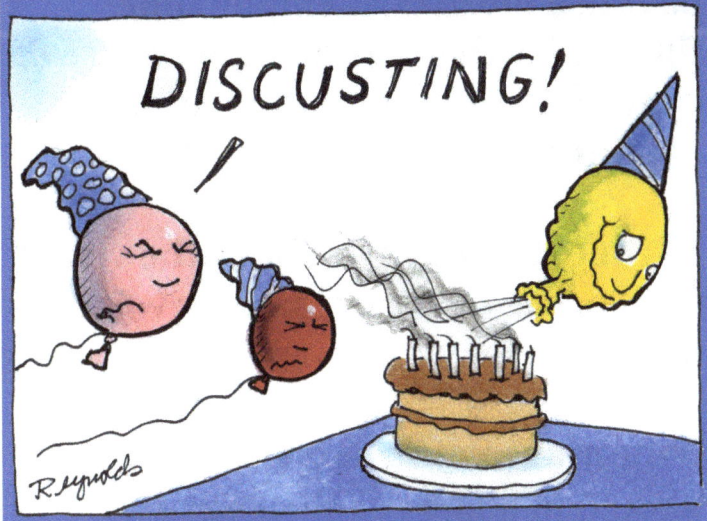

For those wishing to lose weight, the good news with every fart is that you weigh just a little bit less.

Frozen poop stays permanently frozen and does not decompose at high altitude, so there is a growing collection from earlier expeditions to Mount Everest and other summits that is of concern. Climbers are having a more challenging time finding ice that has not been contaminated for melting into drinking water.

The most readily visible of the visual farts occur in the bathtub or when immersed in water.

Over ninety-nine percent of the gas passed in a fart is odorless.

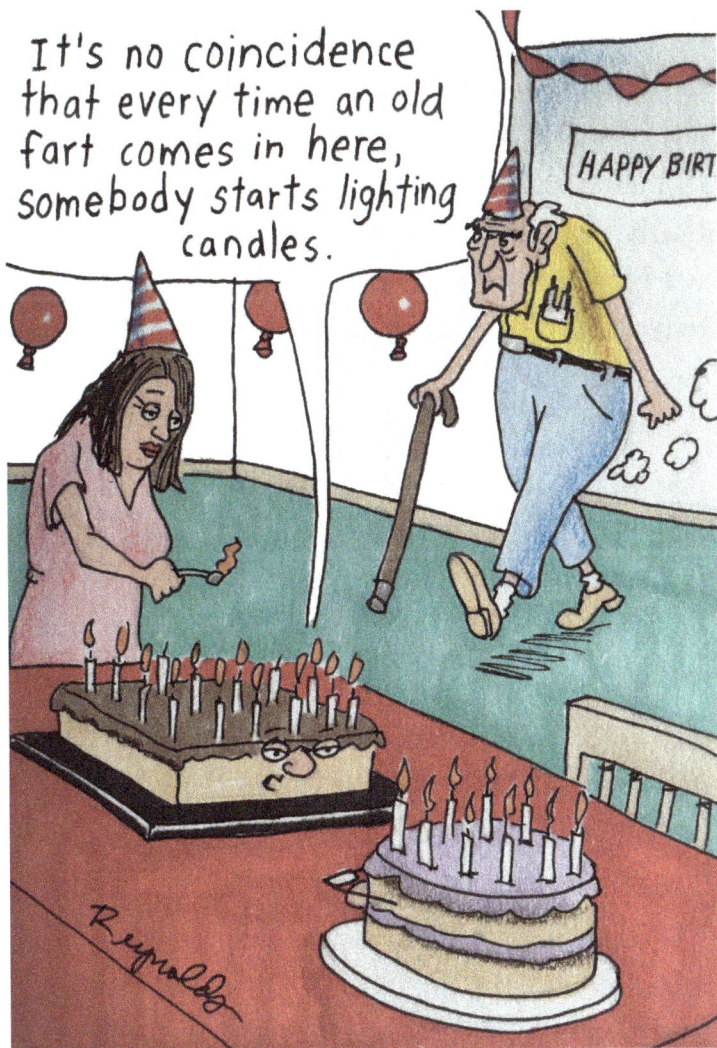

It's no coincidence that every time an old fart comes in here, somebody starts lighting candles.

HAPPY BIRT

Reynolds

As a fart is composed of atoms and molecules it has physical properties, including a mass and weight. Since it is composed of gasses and volatile molecules it is very light, yet the weight is measureable. The total mass of the average fart is 0.0371 grams.

As humans age the production of digestive enzymes decreases so there is a scientific basis for the phrase 'old fart'.

The mechanism of increasing intra-abdominal pressure for a fart is the same as generating increased intra-thoracic pressure for a sneeze. This involves attempted exhalation against a closed epiglottis, and is known as the Valsalva maneuver.

The Fart Side: Life is a Gas!

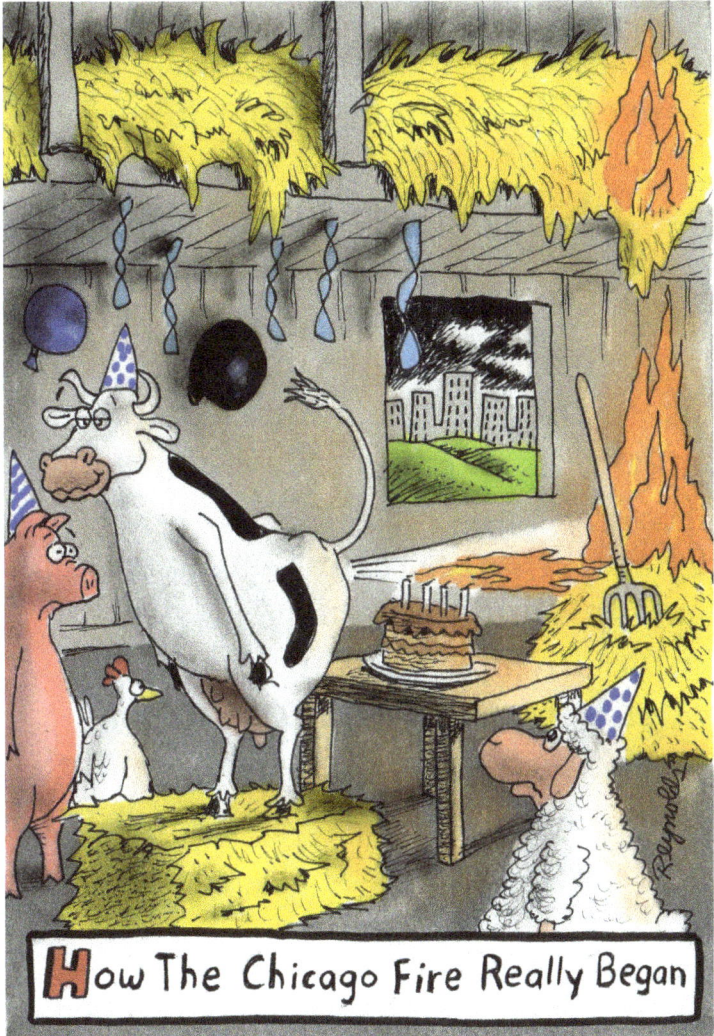

How The Chicago Fire Really Began

Farts have been recorded with the speed of aroma traveling at a conservative ten miles per hour.

English is the richest language with more words than any other.

The word fart is the correct word to use in the English language, and indeed is one of its oldest words.

The alternative terms for a fart, such as flatus and flatulence, are not originally English words as they have been borrowed from the Latin. In Latin, these words have the general meaning of a wind, or a blowing.

Nitrogen bubbles in a beverage are smaller and longer lasting than carbon dioxide bubbles.

The Fart Side: Life is a Gas!

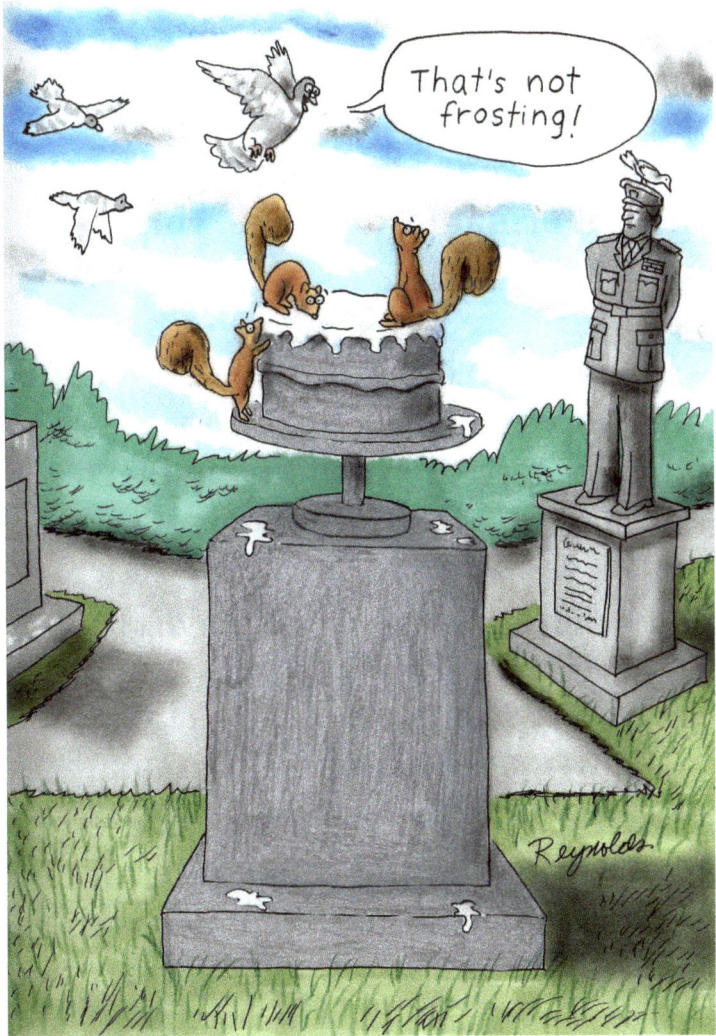

There is controversy as to the derivation of the word fart. It is thought to have Indo-European roots in the Germanic language word *farzen*.

The Indo-European word *perd* means fart, and this led to the Latin word *pedere* the verb form of fart, and *peditum* the noun form of fart.

The related Greek word *perdix* referred to a type of bird that made an explosive fart-like sound when it was flushed from the brush when startled. While being incorporated from Greek to Old French it became *perdriz*, then Middle English *partrich*, and finally Modern English *partridge*.

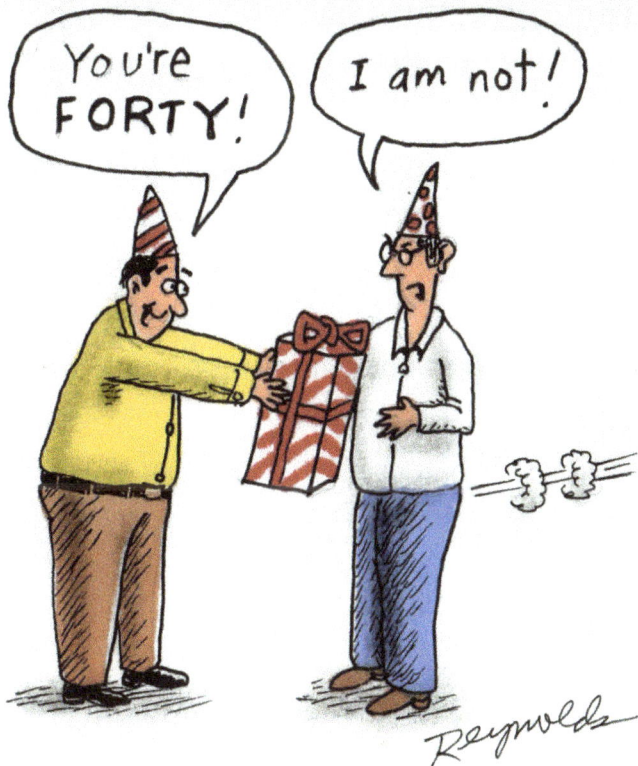

The word fart is also found in other languages, but there it often has a different and unrelated meaning.

In the Scandinavian languages, the word fart usually denotes speed or motion. In Danish and Norwegian, it is often used in combination with other words that obscures the meaning even more.

For example, in Danish a *fartcertifikate* means a trade certificate.

In Norwegian, a *fart plan* means a schedule.

The Norwegian phrase *stå på fartin* pronounced as stop-a–fartin means ready to leave.

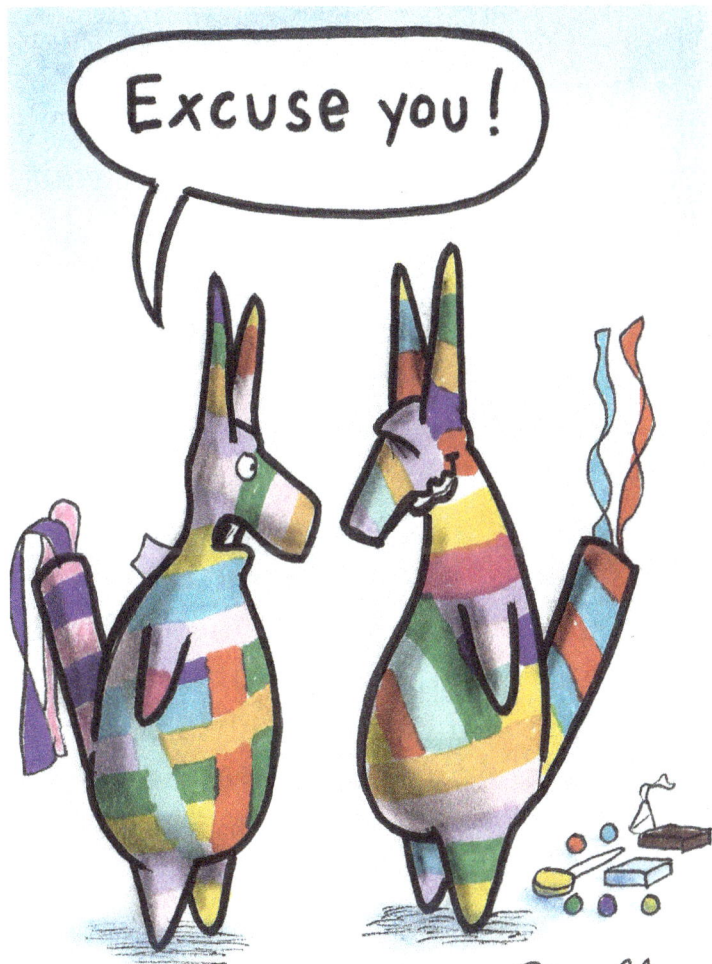

In then Scandinavian languages the phrase *farts måler* pronounced as fart smeller refers to a speedometer.

In Swedish, a speed bump is called a *farthinder*. *Fartlek* is speed training by running at alternate intervals of fast and slow paces.

If you travel on a Scandinavian marine vessel, you may see the control of engine speed labeled as *half-fart* and *full-fart* for half-speed and full-speed respectively. Fart kontrol zones are speed zones.

In Italy, the word *farto* means mattress.

In Hungary, *fartaj* means buttocks.

The Fart Side: Life is a Gas!

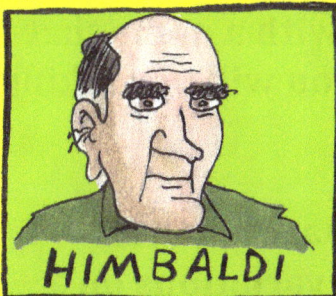
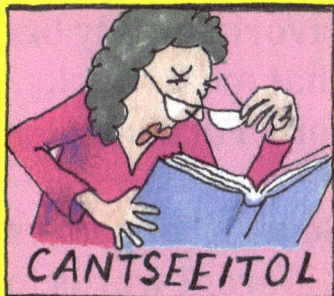
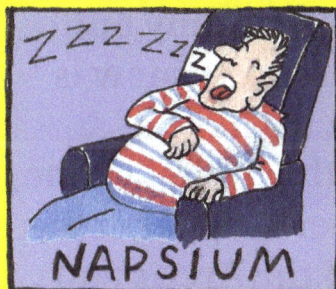
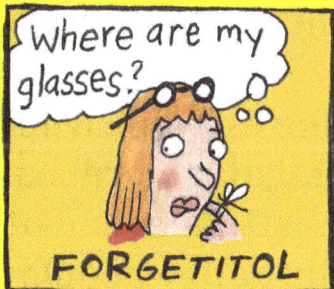
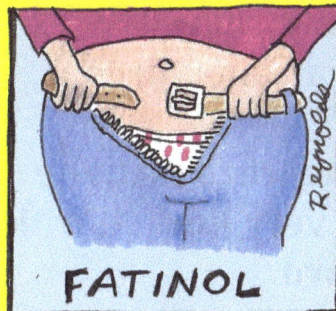
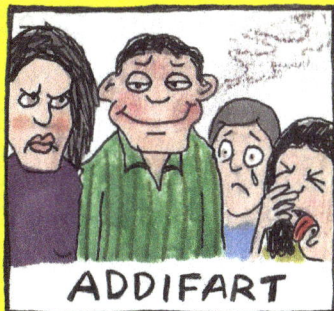

In Poland, if you want to buy a local favorite candy bar with a name that that means lucky, you will be looking for a *Fart* bar.

Several languages have several different words for variations on a theme for which there is only one word in English. The word snow is one example where we have a singular word, but the Inuit, Eskimo, Aleut, Sami and other languages of the native people of the Arctic and northern latitudes may have hundreds of snow variant words.

When it comes to the word fart, the English language is very limited with just the singular word.

The Fart Side: Life is a Gas!

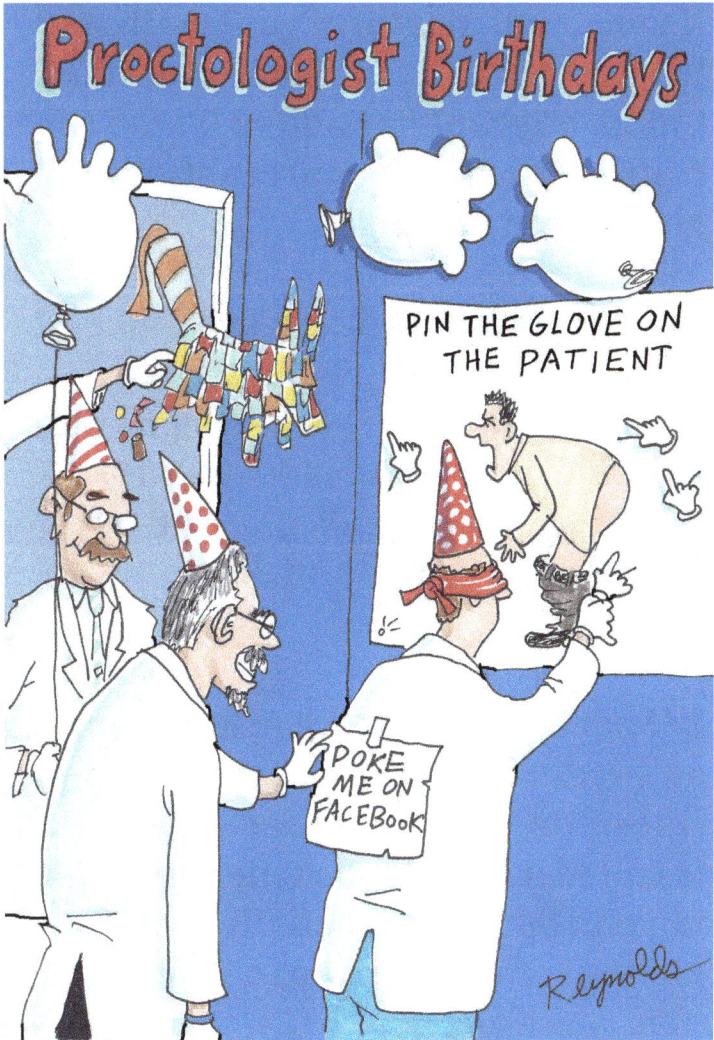

If you smell a natural gas (methane) leak, it is not the methane you smell, but an odorant gas added by the gas company as a safety precaution to give notice of danger.

In Germany, a similar word *fahrt* means a journey, trip, tour, or passage. It is often seen in signs that say e*infahrt* (sounds like in-fart) and *ausfahrt* (sounds like out-fart) denoting entrance and exit respectively.

In Spanish and Portuguese fart means an excess of anything, especially food. One of the richest desserts they offer is called a *farte*, which means a fruit tarte in Spain, and usually a sugar almond or cream cake in Portugal.

The Fart Side: Life is a Gas!

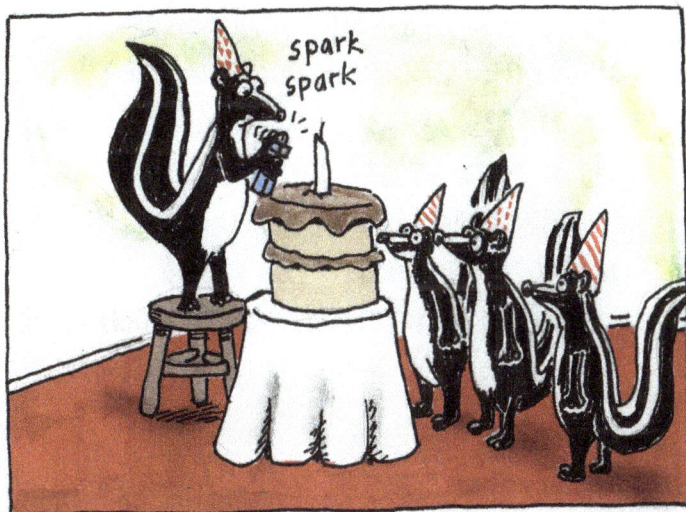

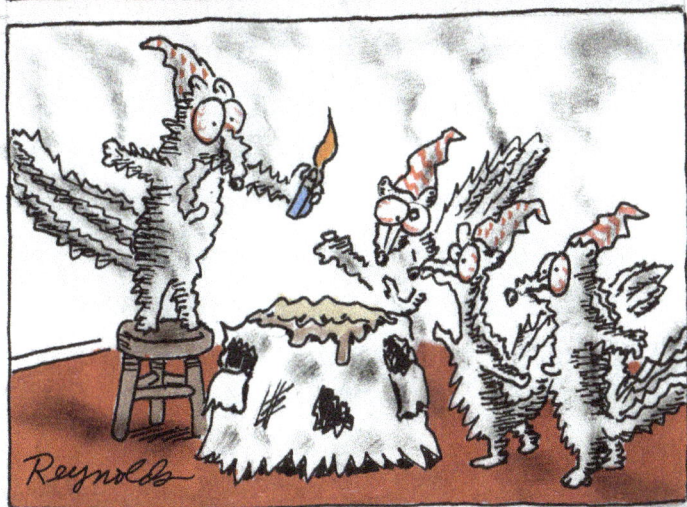

Some of the Russian verbs for the action of farting are particularly colorful. *Perdet'* (to fart with or without sound), *bzdet'* (to fart silently), *pereperdet* (to fart repeatedly), and *nabzdet'sya* (to fart silently to one's complete and utter satisfaction)!

The word fart is one of the oldest words in the English language. One of the most influential dictionaries in the long history of the language is Samuel Johnson's *A Dictionary of the English Language* published in 1755. An important innovation in his dictionary was the use of quotations from literature to illustrate the usage of the word defined.

The Fart Side: Life is a Gas!

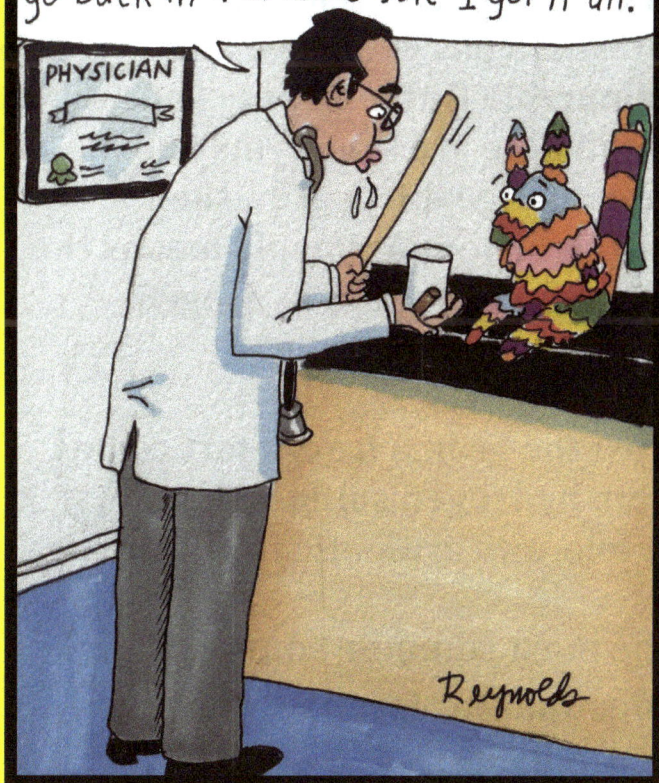

While a minority of individuals may have methane present in their farts, methane is odorless.

The individual gasses that make intestinal gas explosive and flammable (inflammable and flammable are synonyms and interchangeable words, their antonym nonflammable means the exact opposite) are hydrogen, methane, and oxygen.

Most the aroma from a fart comes from hydrogen sulfide, skatole, indole, and aromatic fatty acids.

The most common source of intestinal gas is air swallowing (aerophagia)

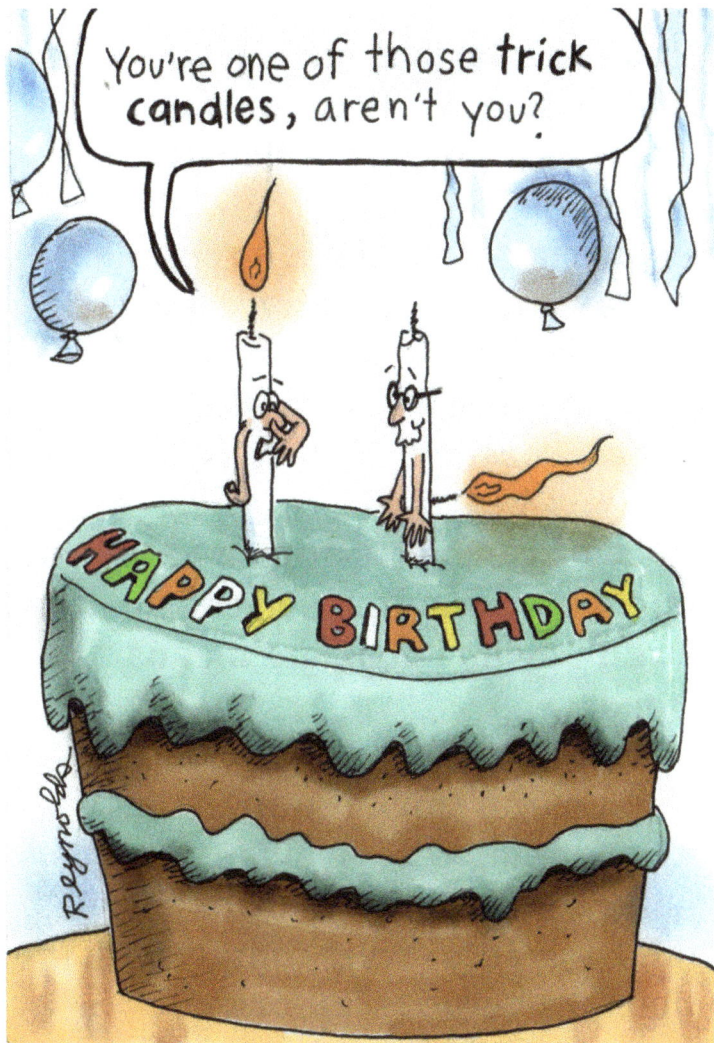

While vegetarians may fart more than carnivores, the aroma is not nearly as pungent or offensive.

Twelve farts per day is a reasonable approximation of the average number of farts humans pass each day, but there is a very wide range of what is considered normal.

The word Fart in northern European languages including German and the Scandinavian languages means speed.

The sense of smell requires that odorant molecules from the source material travel to the nasopharynx and come into direct contact with the olfactory nerve receptors.

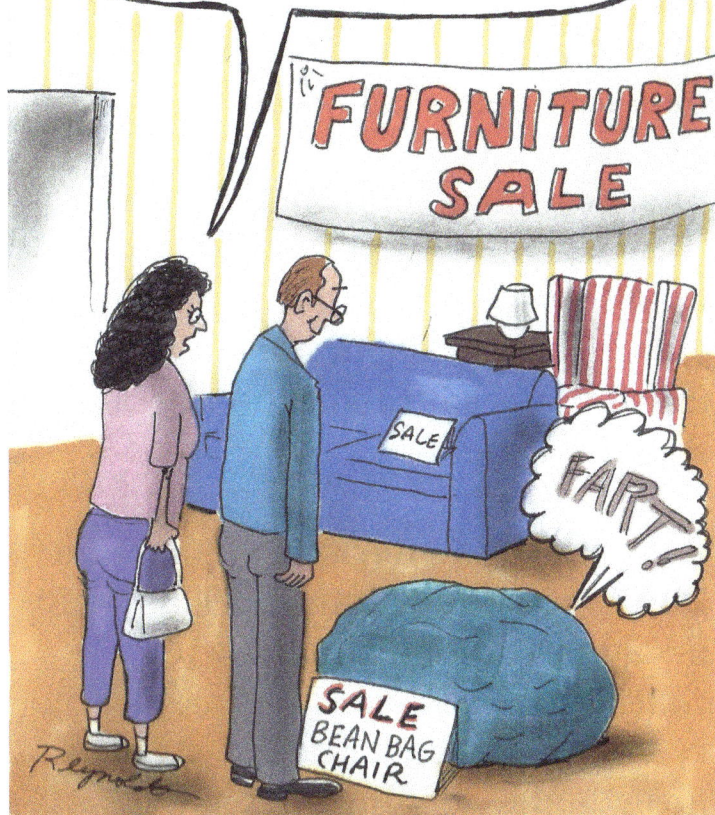

The detection of a fart requires that the odorant molecules that arose in the intestinal tract, and was released as a fart, had to travel all the way to your nose and have direct contact direct with the cilia receptors of your olfactory nerve cell.

A fart contains odorants, as well as transmissible microbes. It is possible to become ill and acquire a pathogen leading to an infection from a fart, much like what can occur with a cough or sneeze.

Pumpernickel (German translation: Devil's Fart) is a heavy dark brown bread traditionally made with coarsely ground rye flour and whole rye berries, which often leads to the intestinal gas giving it its name.

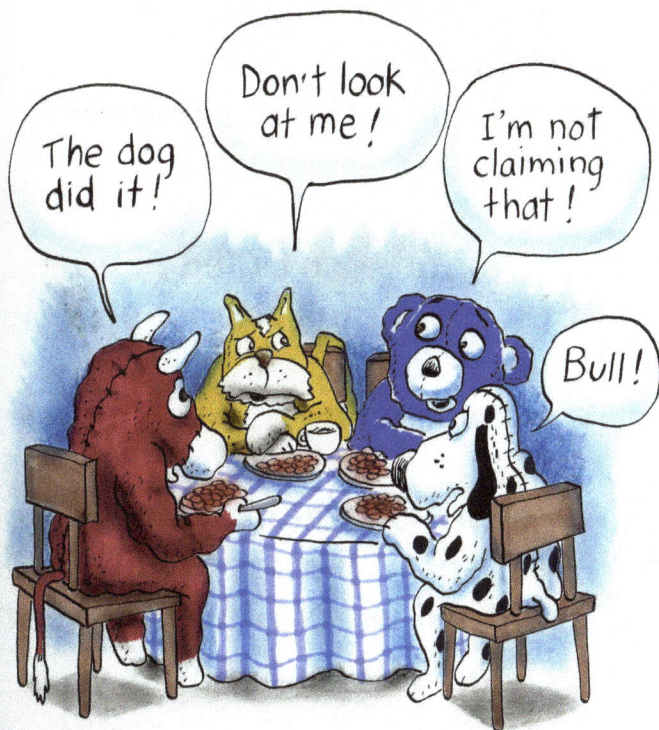

Like most rye breads, pumpernickel is traditionally made with an acidic sourdough starter, which inhibits the rye amylase enzymes.

Without amylase, complex starches such as amylose cannot be metabolized and lead to increased intestinal gas.

Pets de Nonne, also called Pets de Sœur (French translation: nun's farts) are a light airy dessert puff pastry dating from medieval times.

In Western and other cultures, a body may be displayed prior to burial. As the intestinal gas production does not cease with death, and indeed accelerates, gas may continue to escape as an audible fart.

The Fart Side: Life is a Gas!

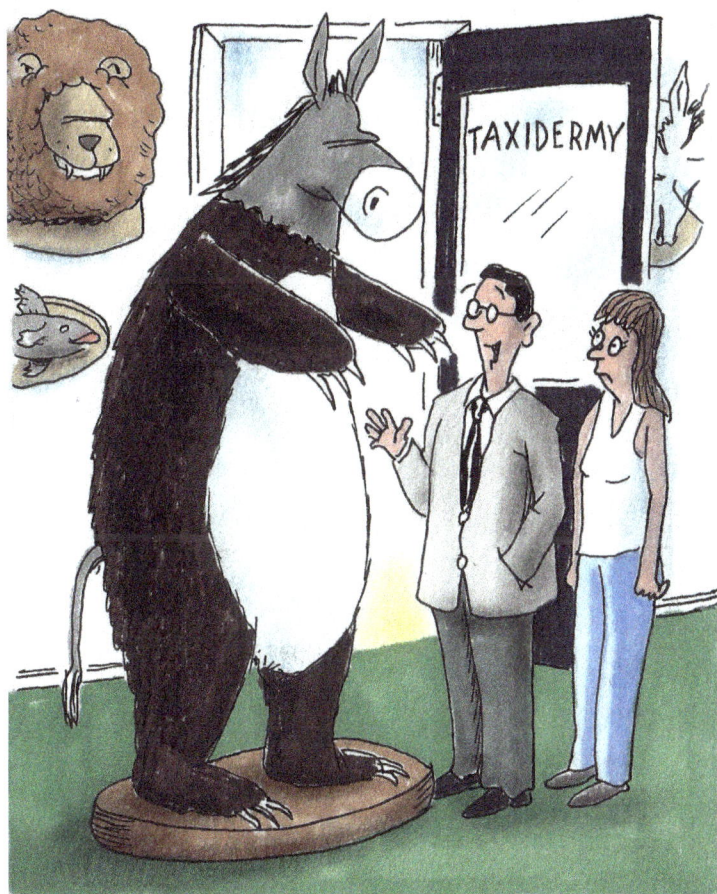

"I don't usually show this on a first date, but I thought you'd like to see my bear-ass."

Part of the mortician practice is to perform a procedure that seals and secures the anus of the deceased so that the audible release of gas does not occur. Many have been frightened that the corpse is alive.

One of the most common causes of excess gaseousness is the deficiency of the enzyme lactase, known as lactose intolerance.

Lactase hydrolyses the complex disaccharide dairy sugar lactose into the readily absorbable simple sugars of glucose and galactose.

Rice is the one starch exception and rarely contributes to significant gas production.

The Fart Side: Life is a Gas!

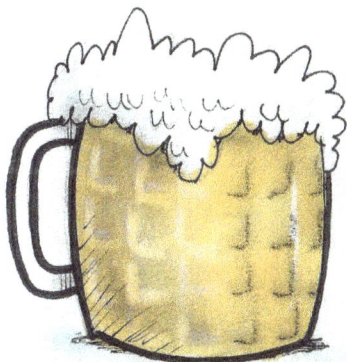

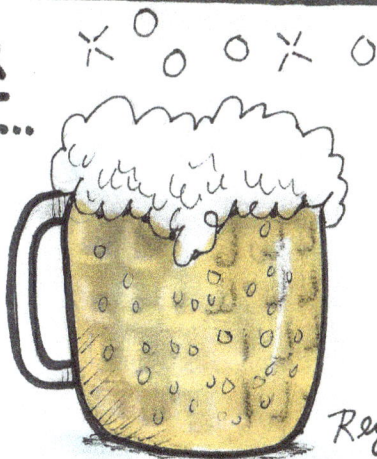

With insufficient lactase, the sugar molecule is not metabolized by the digestive system but is instead metabolized by the gut flora, also known as the microbiome. Lactase deficiency results in gas production and may also give rise to cramps and diarrhea.

Wheat has the other 'distinction' of having the protein glutamate, which contains the nitrogen base product which generates ammonia-like aromatic compounds that contribute to the aroma of intestinal gas

There are many specific enzymes required in the process of digestion, and deficiency in the quantity or activity of an enzyme can lead to food intolerance.

The Fart Side: Life is a Gas!

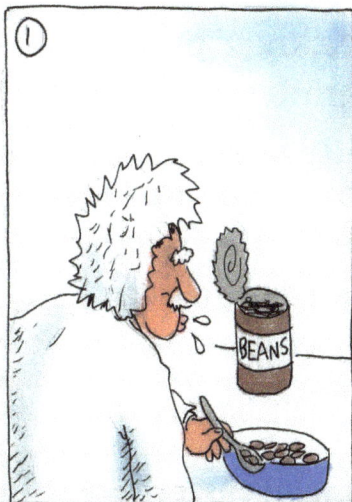

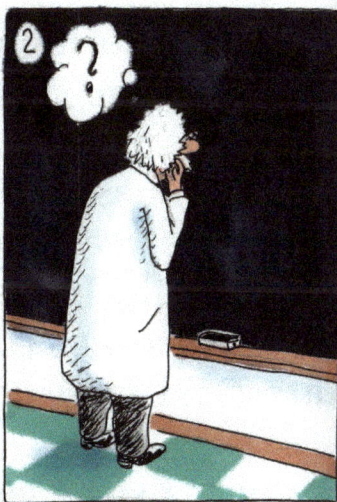

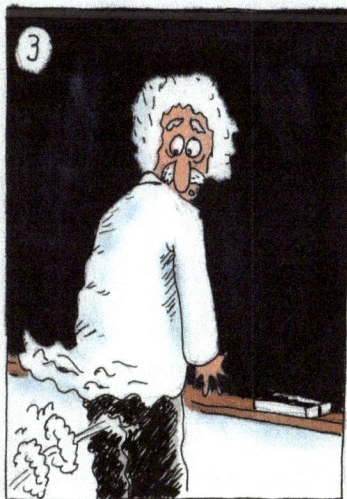

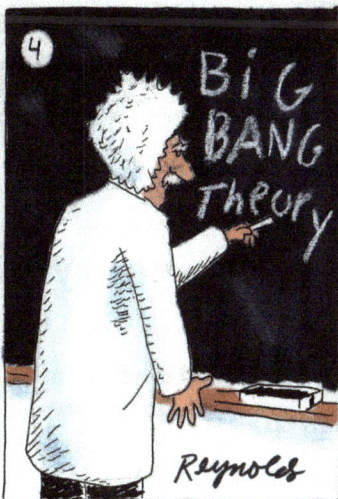

Dozens of hormones, over one thousand and six hundred enzymes, over tens of thousands of species of gut microbes, and over one million genes are just some of the variables effecting the human response to its diet, which also contributes to intestinal gas production.

Air may also be inflated into the colon as the self-practice of the air enema. An air enema is described in the ancient yoga literature as a shake or vat baste.

The advanced yogi may develop anal sphincter control, and control of the abdominal muscles to create an abdominal suction effect to vacuum air into the lower intestine.

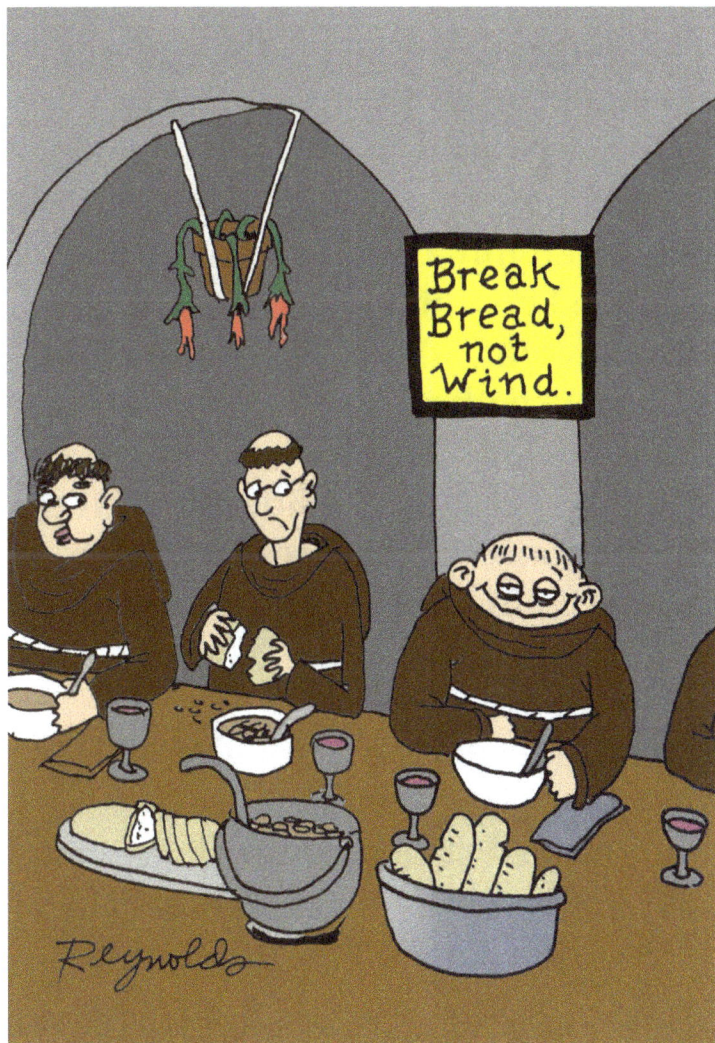

The ability to air fart is the common term for the ability to control the anus and muscles of abdomen and respiration, to cause air to be aspirated into the colon and then released voluntarily as a fart. It is also known colloquially as the ability to butt breathe.

Although usually considered under involuntary control these muscles can be trained, and yogis attain remarkable proficiency.

The air fart and butt breathe technique is known in more enlightened society as an air enema and has been practiced as a part of yoga colon hygiene for thousands of years.

The Fart Side: Life is a Gas!

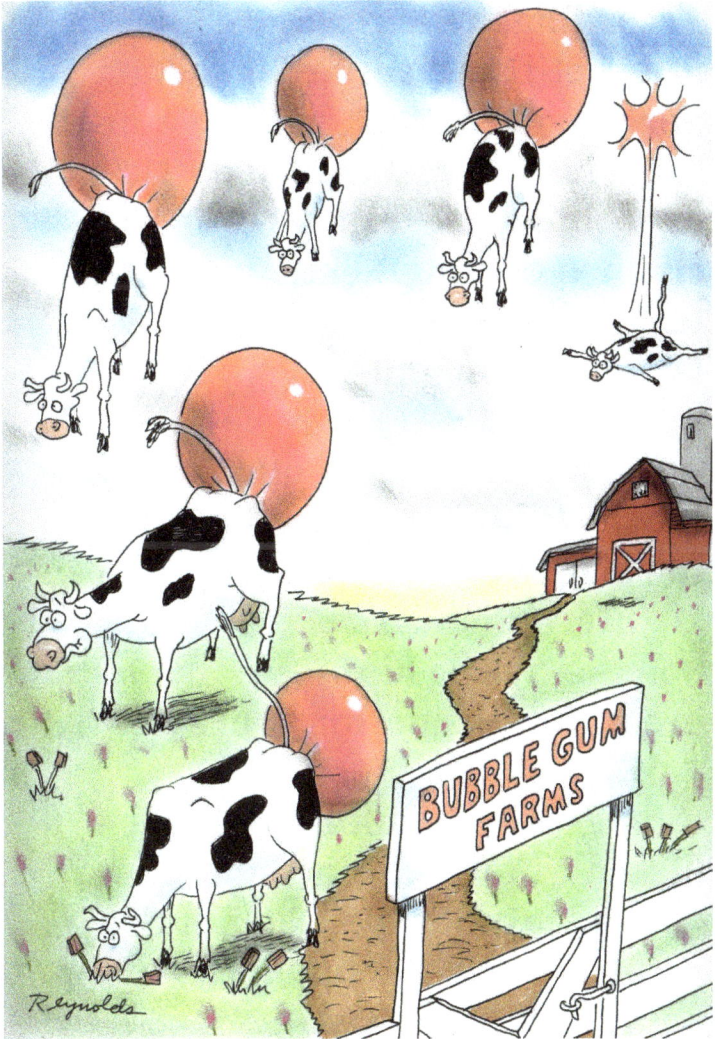

According to the results of an internet-based survey on farting performed in 2001, with over one thousand three hundred participants, over fifteen percent of respondents claimed they could accomplish this task, with the result of being able to fart on command.

At the turn of the twentieth century, the performer Joseph Pujol, under the stage name Le Pétomane, became an international sensation by demonstrating his prowess at butt breathing as a performance art.

It takes several million jasmine blossoms to make one pound of natural jasmine oil, which is two-point-five percent indole, a common odorant found in farts.

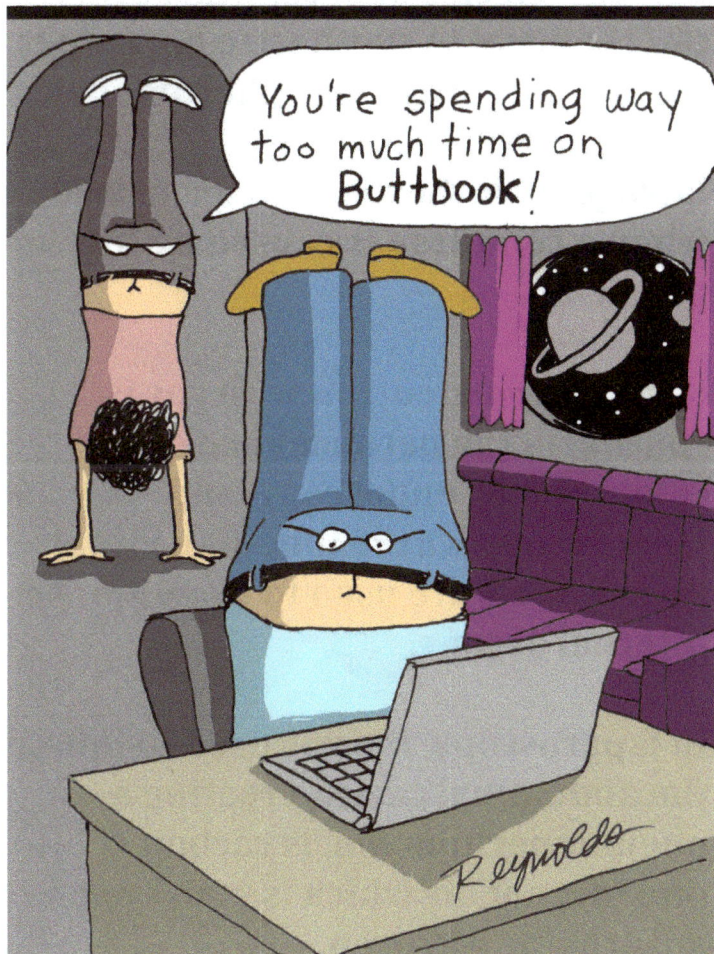

Skatole is attractive to males of various species of bees, who gather the chemical to synthesize hormones that are sex attractant pheromones.

Iatrogenic is the medical term used when a condition is caused by the physician.

Iatrogenic distension with gas is routine in the performance of colonoscopy, endoscopy, and laparoscopy where tube-like visual instruments are used to examine the internal organs.

In laparoscopy, the gas used to inflate the abdominal cavity, creating a pneumoperitoneum, is carbon dioxide, not air which is mainly non-absorbable nitrogen.

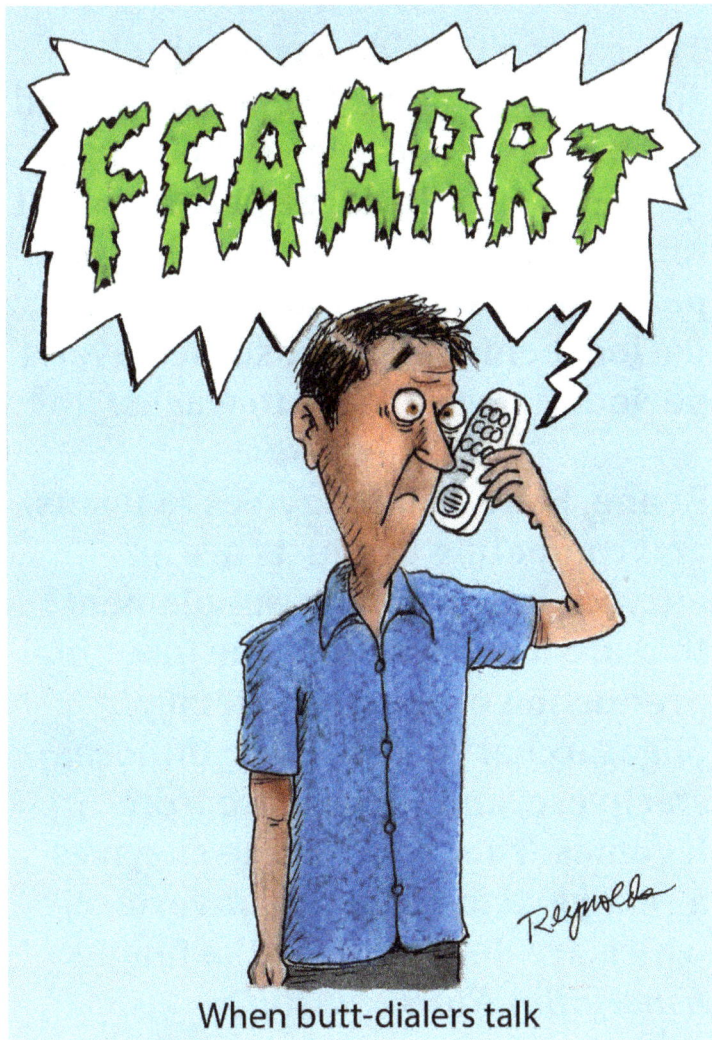

When butt-dialers talk

The carbon dioxide gas is rapidly absorbed by the body and eliminated via exhalation through the lungs. If air were used the large percentage of nitrogen would remain within the peritoneal cavity for an extended period, being slowly absorbed over a period of several days to weeks.

Beano, Bean-Zyme, Say Yes to Beans, and competing products are an enzyme-based dietary supplement that are used to reduce the intestinal production of gas from dietary oligosaccharides such as raffinose, stachyose, and verbascose from legumes. They contain the enzymes alpha-galactosidase and invertase, which are derived from the fungus *Aspergillus Niger*.

The Fart Side: Life is a Gas!

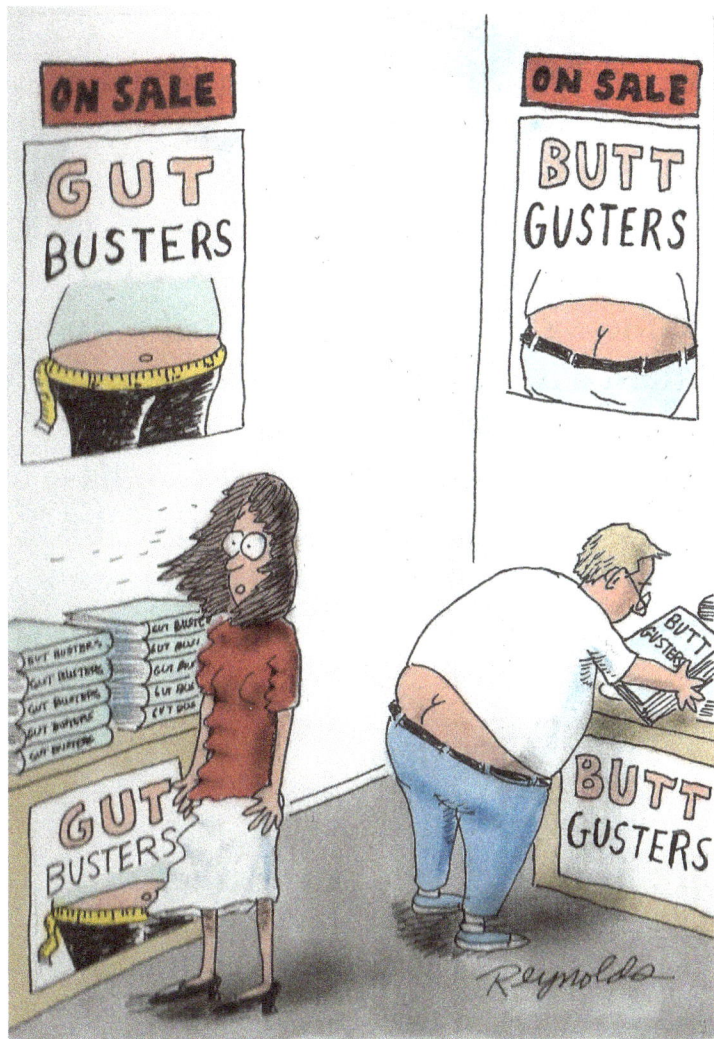

Because pets, such as dogs and cats, also release intestinal gas, the same product was marketed for pets under the brand name Curtail.

Alpha-galactosidase is effective in reducing intestinal gas, but should be taken with the first bite of food.

Because heating inactivates alpha-galactosidase, it is not useful in the cooking process, and must be taken when eating the food. It does not have any effect on lactose or other enzyme deficiencies.

Higher doses of alpha-galactosidase are needed if large quantities of legumes are consumed, or a substantial period has passed since the dose was last taken.

The Fart Side: Life is a Gas!

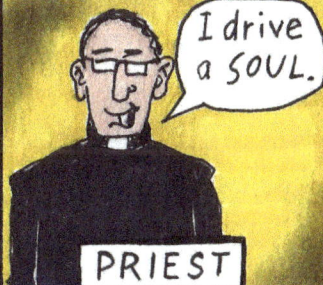
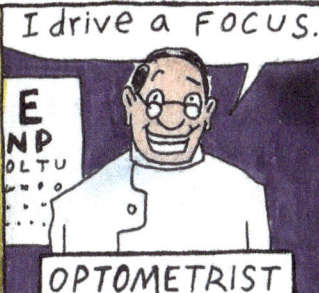
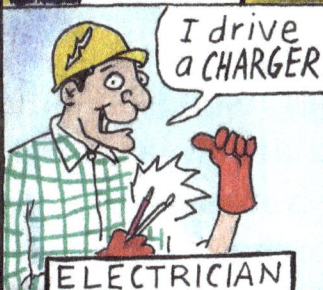
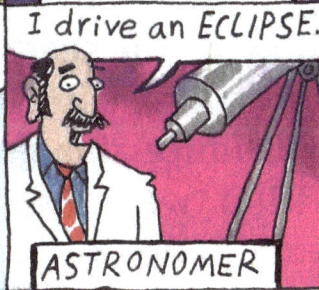

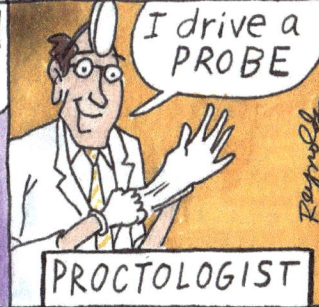

Gas production from legumes can be reduced by soak the beans in water for several hours and discarding the soaking fluid, which leaches out some of the complex sugars.

Most people past more than ten farts per day

Allowing the seeds to germinate allows the bean plant itself to begin to produce alpha-galactosidase. Within twenty-four hours of germination the internally generated enzyme breaks down most of the complex sugars.

Using the herb asafetida can also reduce flatulence, although the herb itself has an aroma that may be worse than the farts that are prevented.

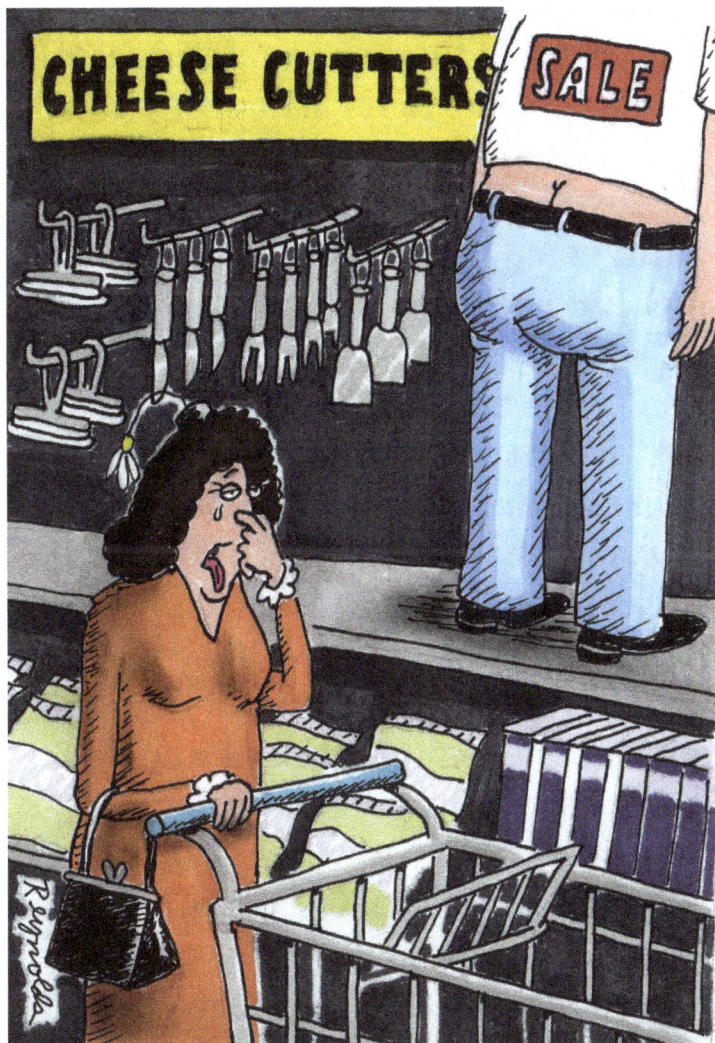

The name of the herb asafetida itself gives a clue as to its aroma. Fetida has the same root as the word fetid. These words are derived from the Latin word *foetidus* and *foetēre* meaning 'to stink'.

Beans are being developed that have lower concentrations of complex sugars. The alpha galactosidase enzyme hydrolyses the complex sugars of the raffinose family including stachyose, verbascose, and galactinol. These are found in foods such as the legumes beans and peanuts, and the cruciferous vegetables cauliflower, broccoli, cabbage, and Brussels sprouts. These complex sugars are the reason the bean is known as 'the musical fruit'.

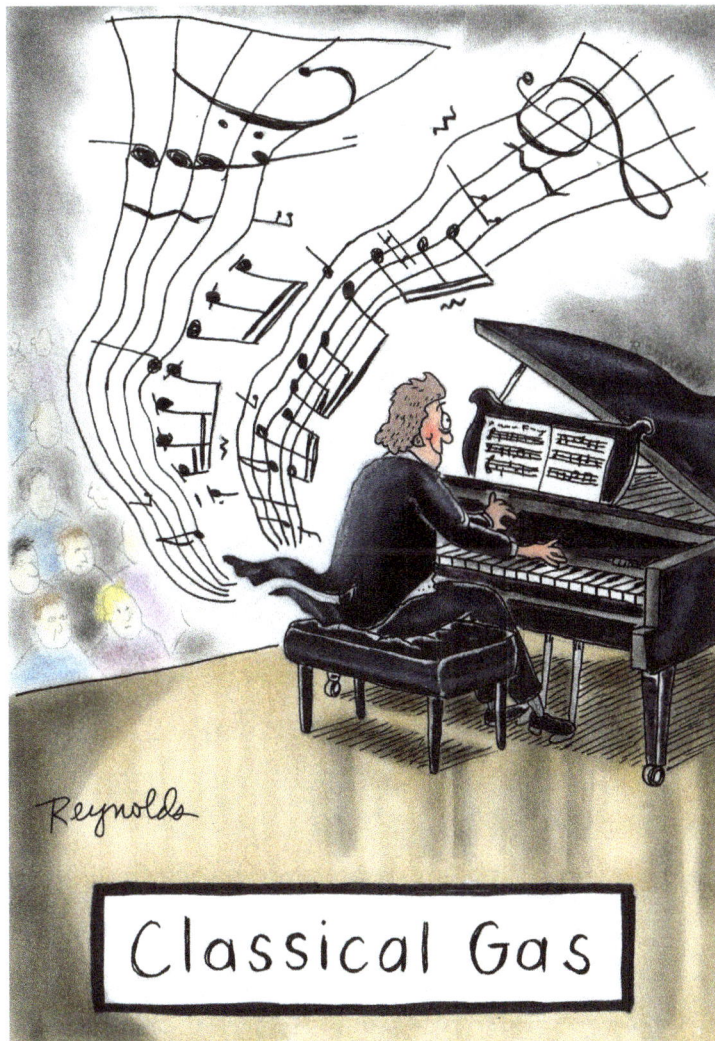

Classical Gas

Beano was marketed by Alan Kligerman of AkPharma, Inc. in 1990. Originally in the dairy farm business, he was the developer of the commercially successful lactase supplement Lactaid. Beano received a US patent in 1995, which has now expired. There are more than fifty competing products on the market. It should be noted that the use of these products enhances the digestibility of certain foods, and increases the nutrients and calories absorbed.

The intellectual concept for a product to reduce intestinal gas was first proposed in the 1780's by the American statesmen, philosopher, humorist, and scientist Benjamin Franklin. He proudly authored an essay entitled 'Fart Proudly'.

The Fart Side: Life is a Gas!

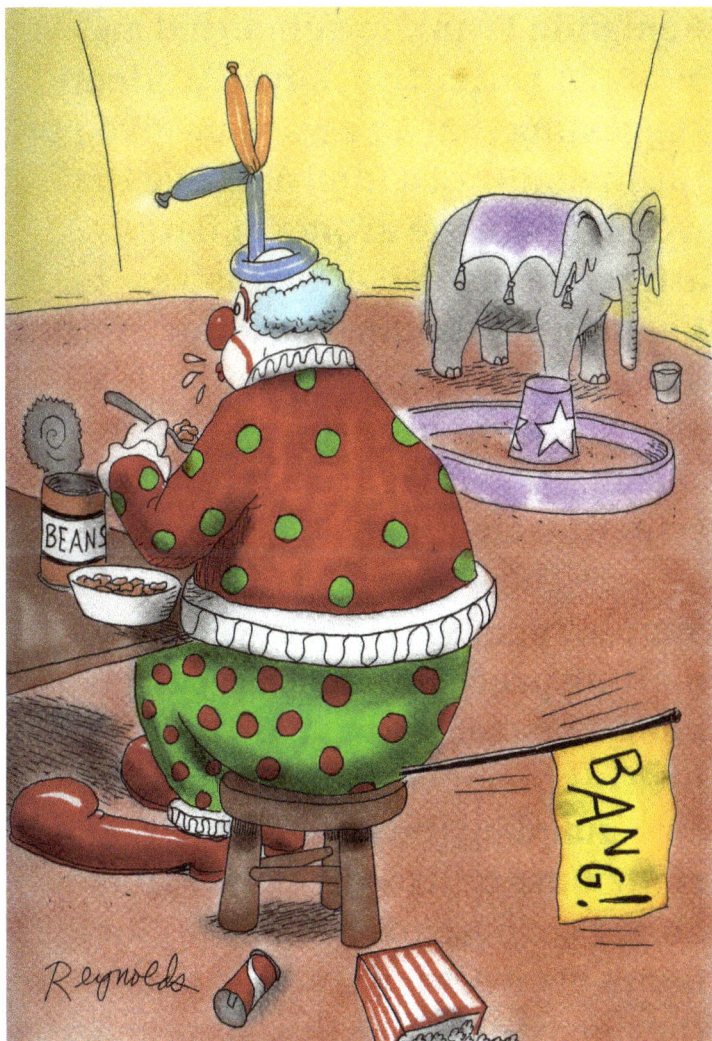

Benjamin Franklin submitted an essay "A Letter to A Royal Academy" suggesting that an award be given to the inventor of a food additive that would make the aroma of flatus attractive instead of offensive. Benjamin Franklin was known as for his sense of humor, and although some thought his proposal was serious, it was written as a satire of scientific meetings.

Simple sugars are produced in the malting process of barley to brew beer. The complex sugars not hydrolyzed or fermented, and thus consumed by the beer drinker, may contribute to its well-recognized ability to increase flatulence. Some home brewers have added Beano to the mash to reduce this occurrence.

The Fart Side: Life is a Gas!

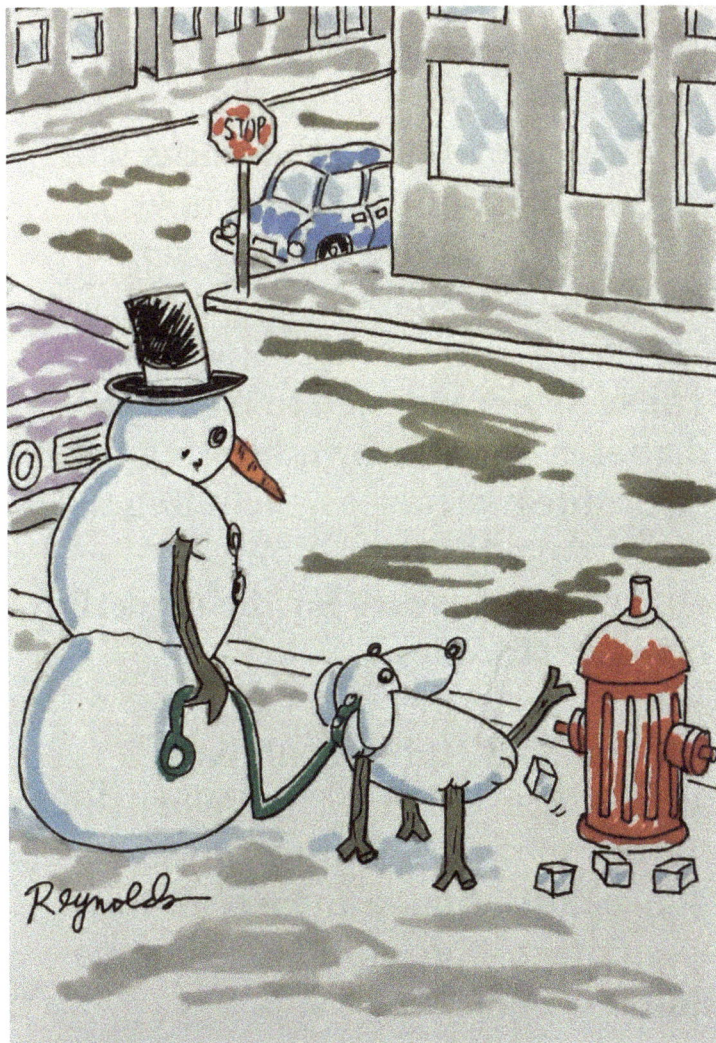

The use of the prescription drug Acarbose or Miglitol used in the treatment of diabetes mellitus will cause a dramatic increase in flatulence because of its enzyme inhibitor activity.

These drugs are used to treat type 2 diabetes mellitus by inhibiting the glycoside hydrolases, including the alpha-galactosidase family of enzymes necessary for the digestion of many starches.

It specifically inhibits alpha-glucosidase enzymes in the brush border of the small intestines, pancreatic alpha-amylase, maltase, isomaltase, glucoamylase, sucrose, and invertase.

The Fart Side: Life is a Gas!

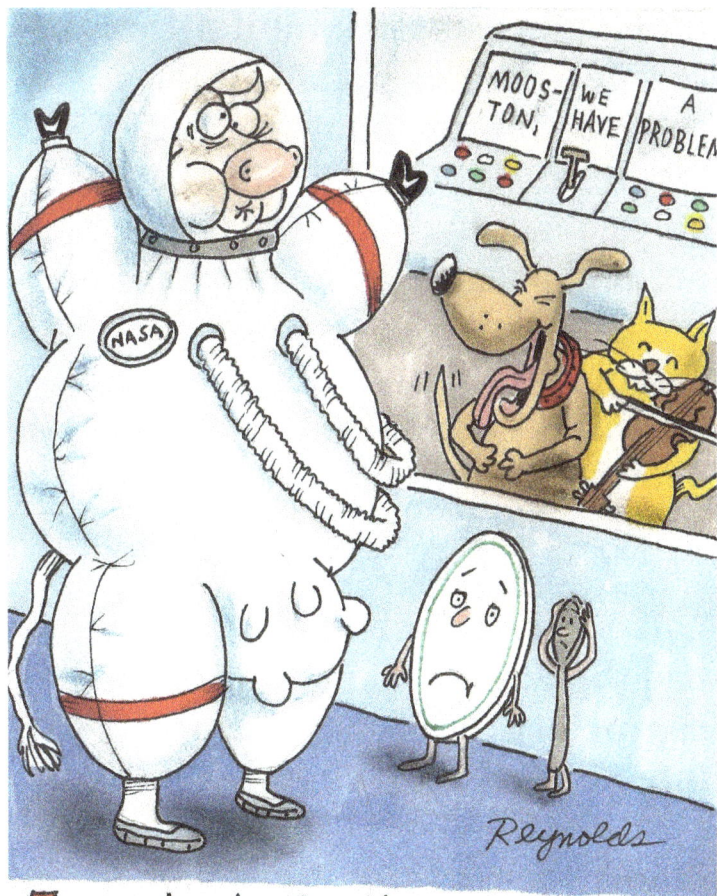

Early tests for the cow's moon jump failed due to faulty equipment and methane gas.

Alpha-glucosidase inhibitors are the competitive, reversible inhibitors of pancreatic alpha-amylase and membrane-bound intestinal alpha-glucosidase hydrolase enzyme. Use of these drugs leads to blockage of the enzymatic degradation of complex carbohydrates in the small intestine, decreasing the amount and delaying the absorption of these sugars.

A diet rich in the amino acid tryptophan can contribute to the characteristic fecal aroma of intestinal gas.

Indole occurs naturally in human feces and contributes to the characteristic fecal odor. Indole is also found in the scent of flowers.

The Fart Side: Life is a Gas!

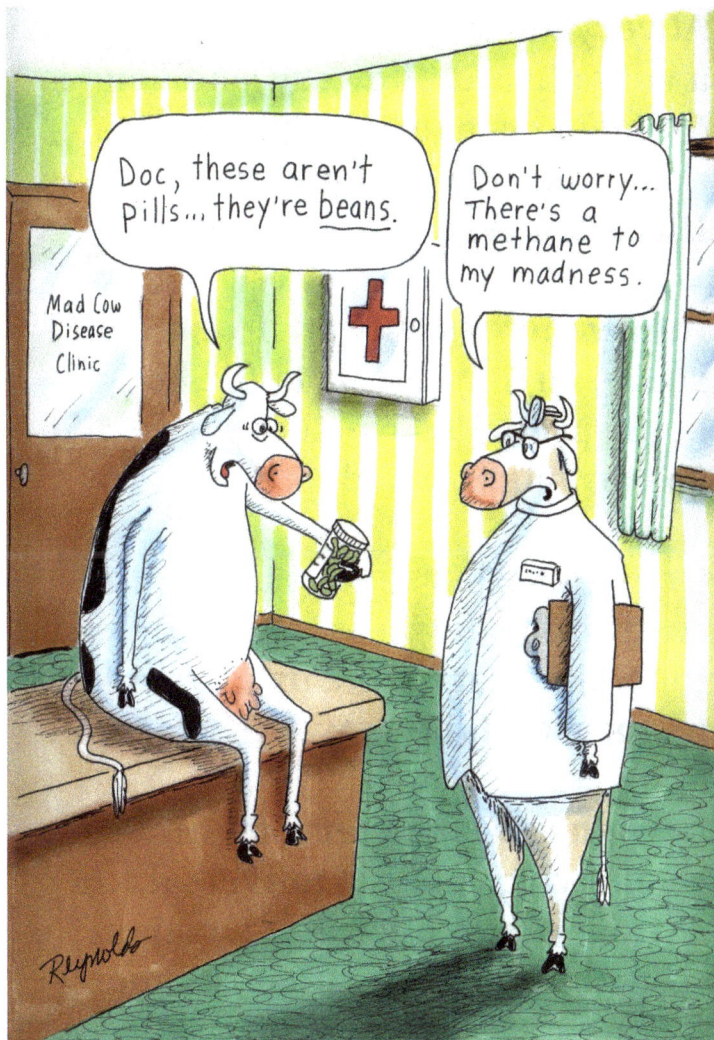

At very low concentrations indole has a very pleasant flowery smell and is found in orange blossoms, jasmine, and other flowers and essential oils. It is often used in perfumes.

In the microgravity environment of space, farting results in the body being propelled when the 'digestive gas thruster is fired'.

On the Russian space station Mir, restraining devices were installed on the toilet seat, so the user would not be thrust off the seat with a fart.

Aerophagia is the term for air swallowing, and is a universal and regular occurrence. It is a major contributor to intestinal gas and farting.

The Fart Side: Life is a Gas!

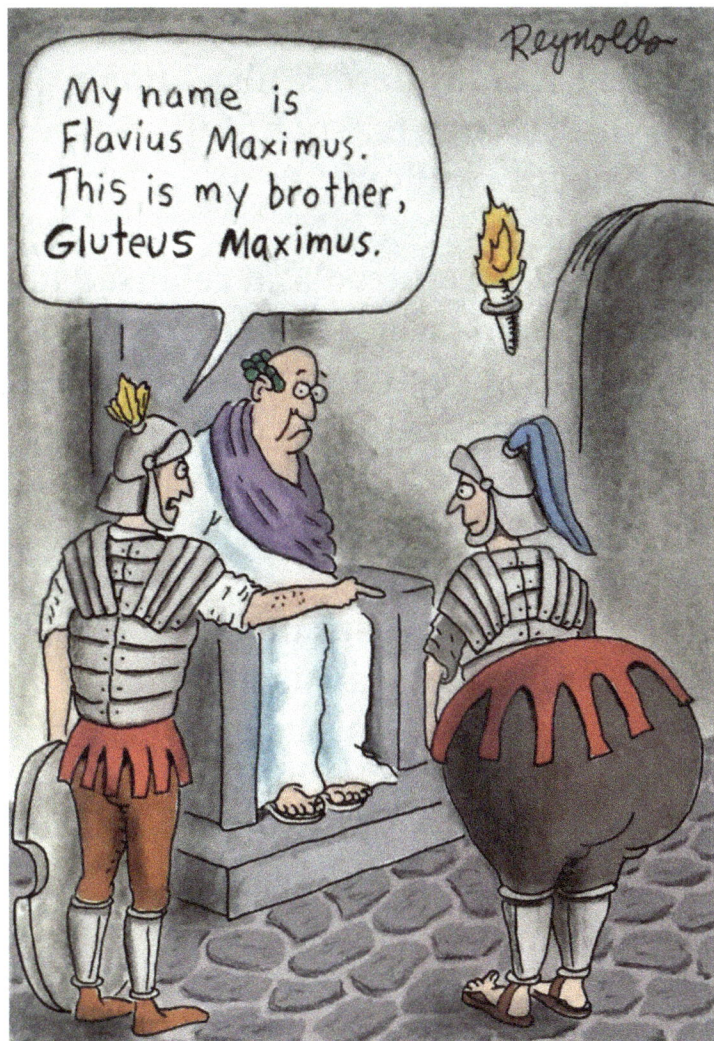

Humans swallow on average three to five cubic centimeters, also known as milliliters, (one teaspoonful) of air with every swallow.

Gasses are produced and released in the gastrointestinal tract during the enzymatic digestive processes as well as the neutralization of gastric hydrochloric acid by pancreatic and duodenal bicarbonate.

The volume of gasses in the gastrointestinal tract is dependent on the quantity and nature of foods ingested, the body's ability to produce enzymes for the various foods consumed, air swallowing (aerophagia), the microbiome and gut flora, and gastrointestinal motility and transit time.

The Fart Side: Life is a Gas!

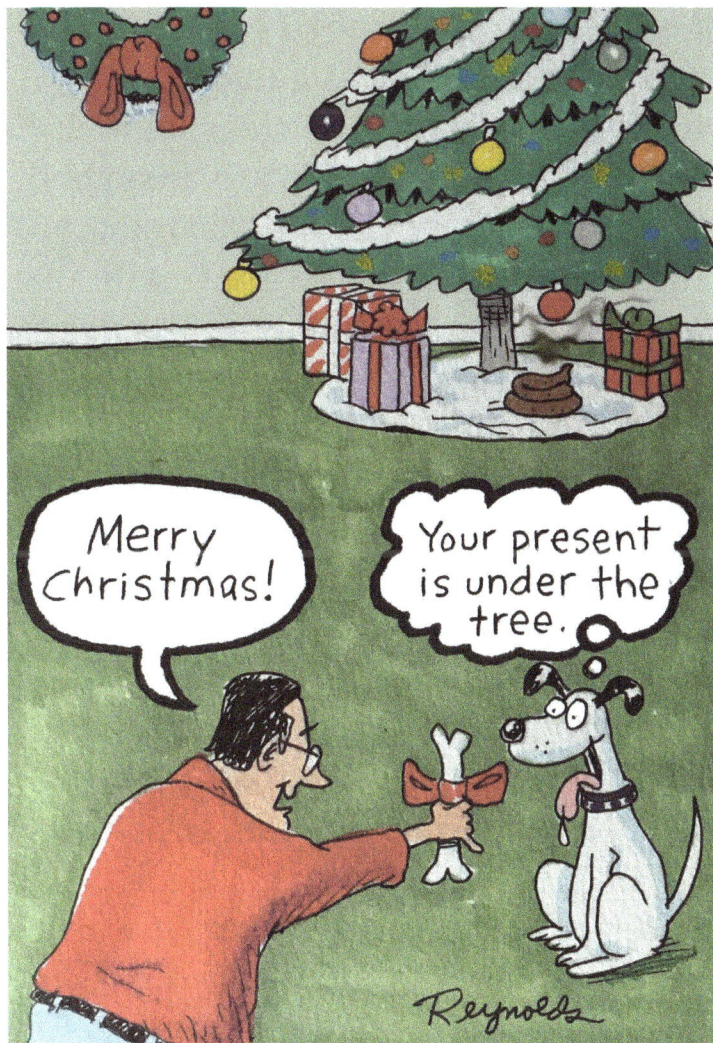

A significant volume of gas is swallowed as well as generated within the bowel. The clear majority of the gasses produced are absorbed by the gut, enter the bloodstream through diffusion, and are finally exhaled when the blood flow reaches the capillaries in the alveoli of the lungs. In the alveoli, the gasses diffuse into the air to be exhaled.

Each of the different component gasses have unique properties of diffusion through the bowel wall and into the bloodstream. Carbon dioxide readily diffuses, and enters and exits the bloodstream in solution easily. Nitrogen has a very difficult time diffusing through the gut wall, and explains why air swallowing leads to distension and bloating.

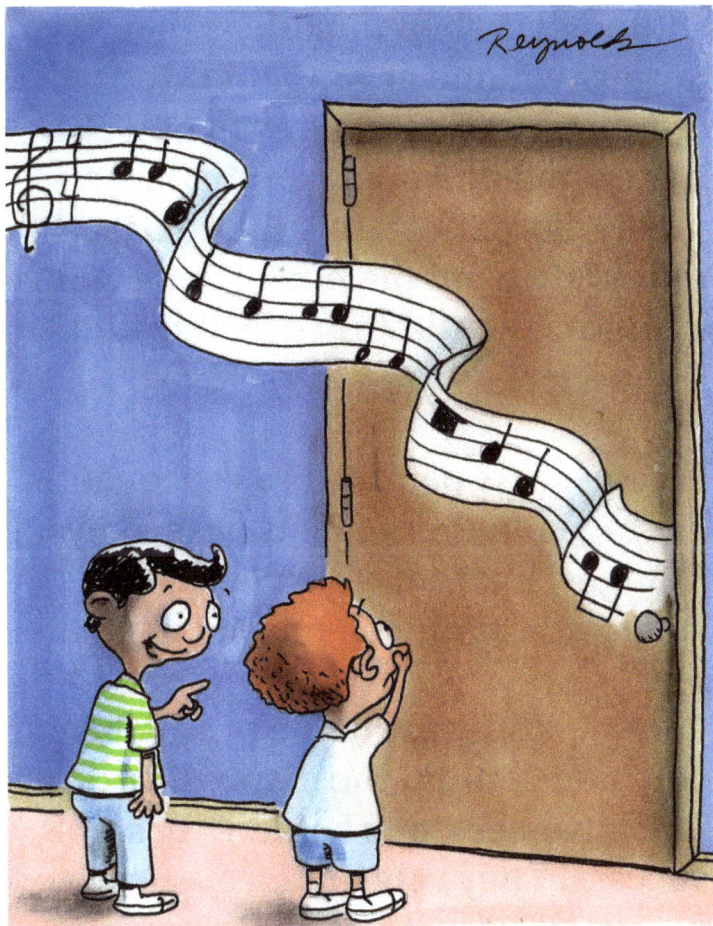

"That's my Dad. He does his best work in the bathroom."

Although carbon dioxide is the largest volume of gas generated, and temporarily contributes to bowel distension and postprandial (after meal) discomfort, it is the easiest to eliminate from the bowel and is only a minor contributor to farting and flatulence.

Twelve farts per day is a reasonable average number of farts passed by humans, but there is a very wide range of what is considered normal.

Commercially available products to trap and contain the dispersion of a fart have been marketed with some success. They rely on the adsorptive properties of activated carbon, also known as activated charcoal, or carbo activatus.

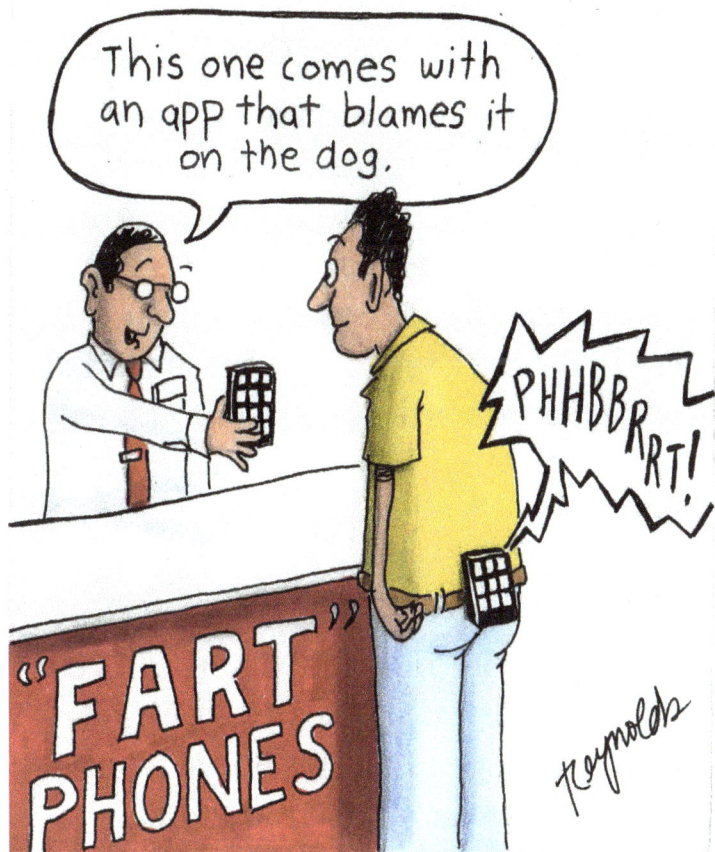

Activated charcoal is a form of carbon processed to increase the surface area available for adsorption or chemical reactions.

Activated carbon is used in the purification, decaffeination, metal extraction, water purification, and sewage treatment processes. It is also used in the air filters in masks and respirators, filters in compressed air, and to filter vodka and whiskey to remove impurities that would affect taste.

Activated charcoal has also been used in cases of the ingestion of toxins or poisons. It is taken orally to bind to the toxin to prevent its absorption from the gastrointestinal tract.

The Fart Side: Life is a Gas!

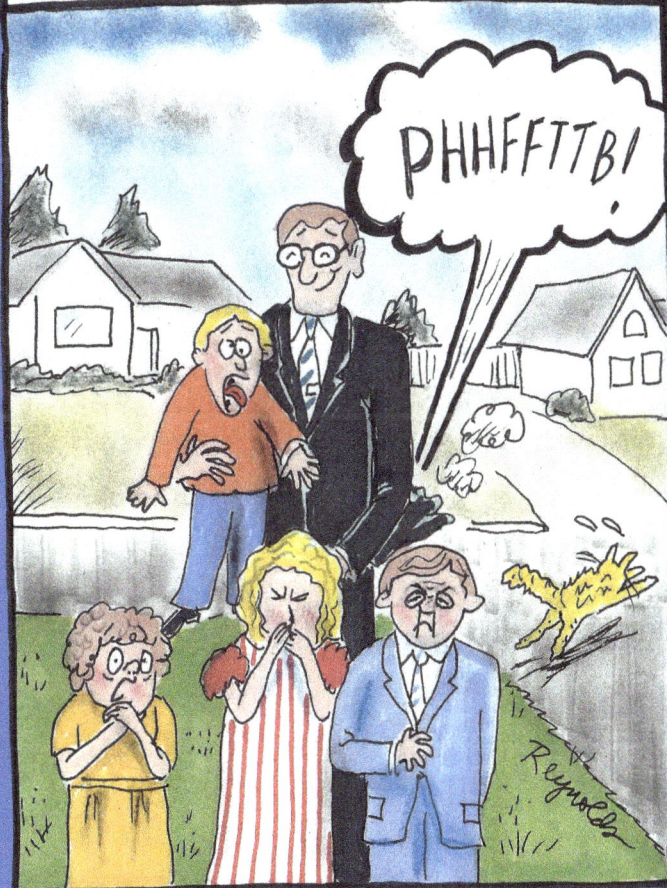

The home remedy of eating burnt toast for food poisoning was based on the adsorptive properties of activated charcoal.

Activated charcoal is also effective in adsorbing offensive smelling gasses in a fart. Due to its porosity, a single gram of activated carbon can have a surface area more than 500 meters squared, with 1500 meters squared being possible with further refining.

Its adsorption ability varies amongst gasses and liquids, and it is known to be a poor adsorbent of carbon monoxide, which is toxic and odorless. It is particularly effective in adsorbing most of the volatile odoriferous gasses of a fart.

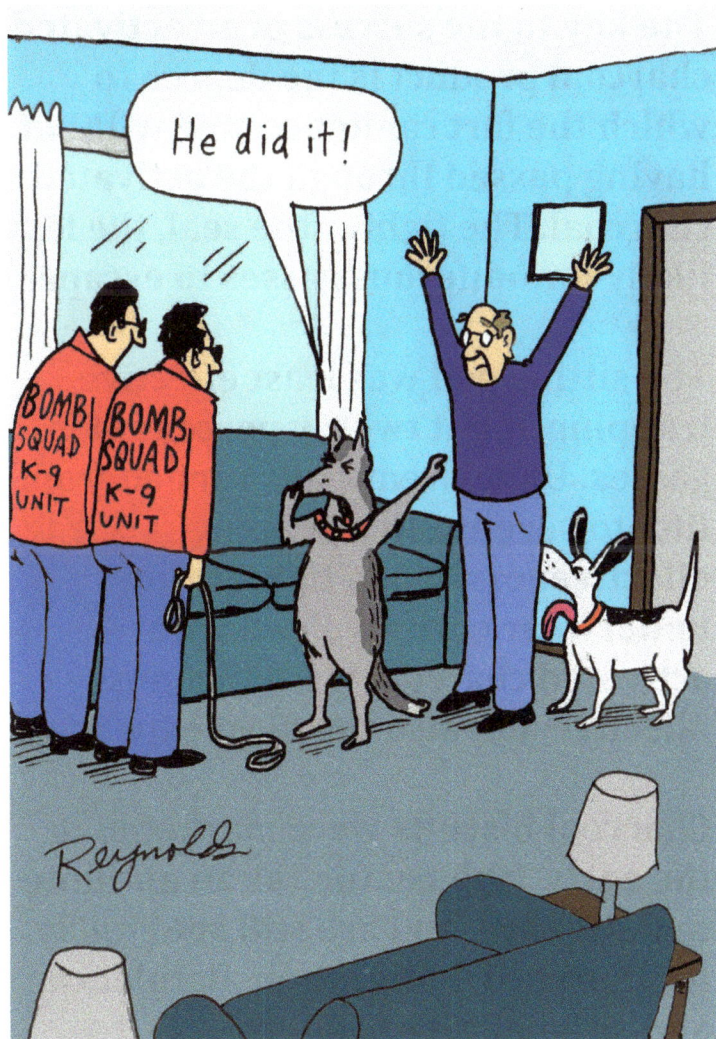

The key to the success of an activated charcoal product is the degree to which the fart cannot escape without having passed through the activated charcoal. The tighter the seal, the less likely for odiferous gasses to escape.

The sitting pad was least effective, trapping about twenty percent of gasses. Underwear pads ranged from fifty to seventy-five percent effectiveness, while tight fitting underwear entirely lined with activated charcoal were the most effective, but also the most expensive.

Charcoal biscuits were marketed in the early 19th century as an antidote to flatulence, and are still sold today for diarrhea, indigestion, flatulence, and as a pet care product.

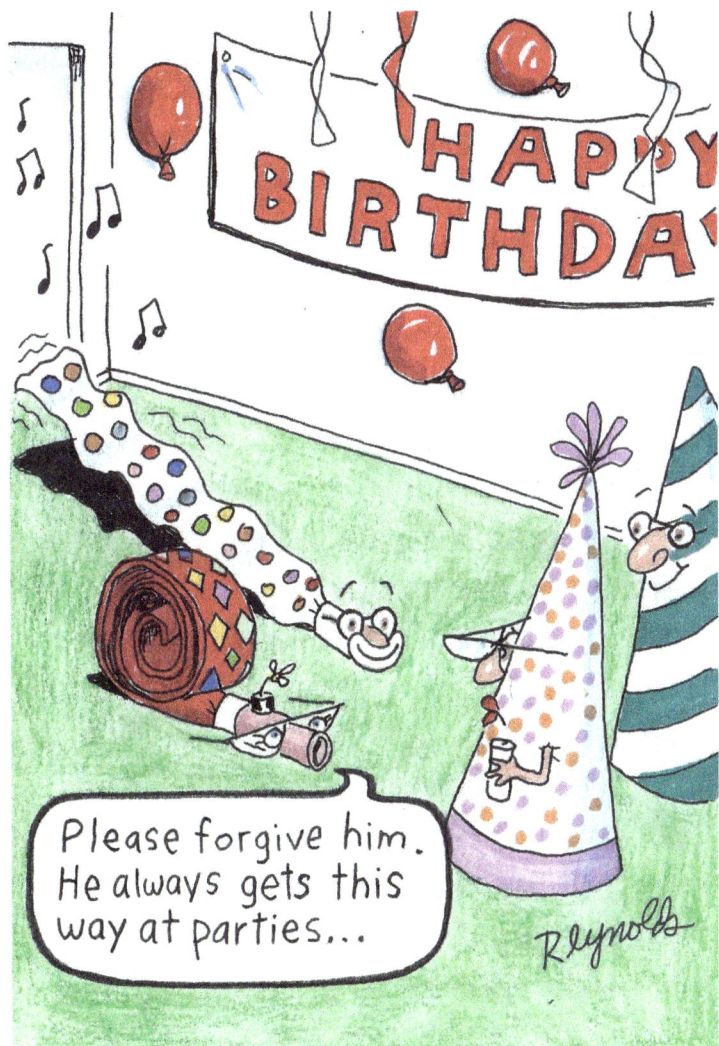

Please forgive him. He always gets this way at parties...

Reynolds

Unfortunately, orally ingested charcoal pills are not as effective in appreciably reducing intestinal gas. This may be because the adsorptive capacity of the activated charcoal is fully utilized before it finally gets to the colon, where its gas adsorbing properties are most needed.

Fortunately, bismuth products do provide a significant advantage by binding to the odiferous sulfur compounds, and preventing them from contributing their offensive odor.

The sulfur hydrogen functional group may also be referred to as a thiol group or a sulfhydryl group. Thiols are also referred to as mercaptans.

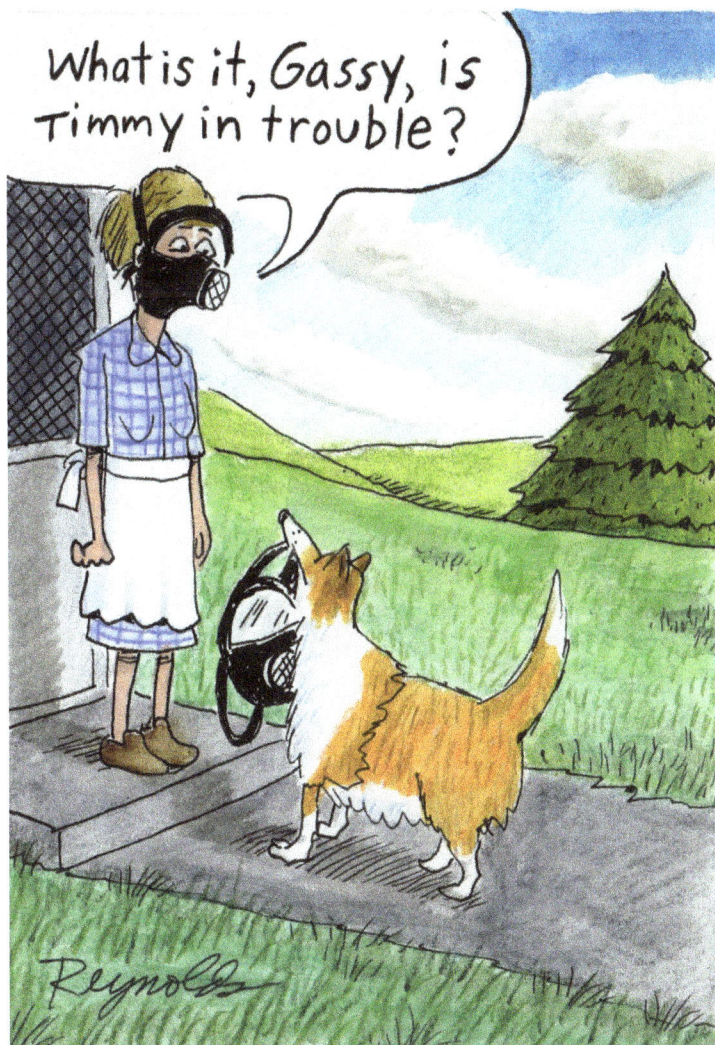

The term mercaptan (Latin meaning 'capturing mercury') is used because the thiolate group bonds so strongly with mercury compounds.

The bacteria of your colonic flora generate gas which collect in the bowel. They are joined with the air swallowed throughout the day and night, particularly at meals.

The word fart may have originated as an onomatopoeia, a word that phonetically imitates the sound of the event it describes.

It may also have been derived from the word partridge as the bird makes similar sound when it is disturbed in its natural habitat and takes flight.

The Fart Side: Life is a Gas!

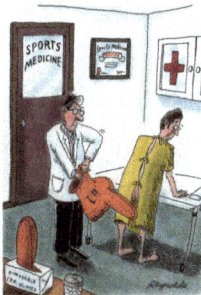

The Fart Side

Blowing in the Wind!

Dan Reynolds
Joseph Weiss, MD

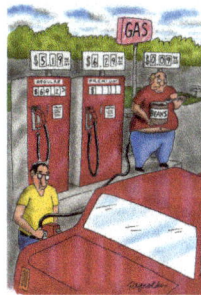

The Fart Side

Life is a Gas!

Dan Reynolds
Joseph Weiss, MD

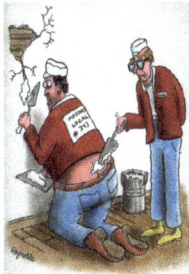

The Fart Side

Bottoms Up!

Dan Reynolds
Joseph Weiss, MD

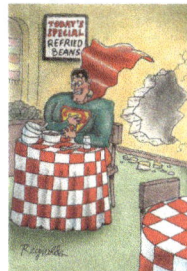

The Fart Side

Windbreaks!

Dan Reynolds
Joseph Weiss, MD

Available in 5"x7" (96 pages) Pocket Rocket! and
6"x9" (122 pages) Expanded Full Blast! editions

www.thefunnysidecollection.com

The Funny Side Collection

Dan Reynolds

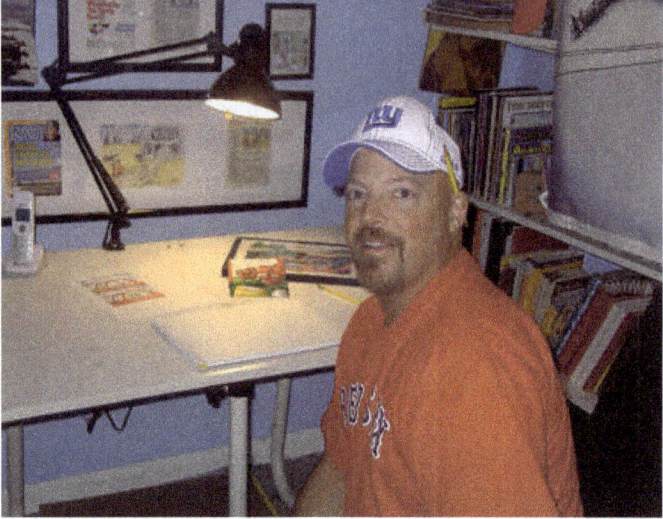

Dan Reynolds began drawing cartoons in December of 1989. He draws and eats left-handed. He plays ping pong and pool left-handed. He throws, kicks and bats right-handed. Like a box of chocolates, you never know what you're going to get, but you will like most of them and they'll keep you coming back. Unlike chocolates, REYNOLDS UNWRAPPED cartoons are not fattening.

Dan's cartoons are seen by millions of readers across the U.S., Canada, and points beyond all the way down under in Australia. His work is seen in every issue of Reader's Digest (where he is known for his cow, pig, and chicken cartoons).

The Fart Side: Life is a Gas!

His cartoons have appeared on HBO's The Sopranos, the cover of a National Lampoon cartoon book collection, and on greeting cards all throughout the United States. His work also appears in many other places as well.

Sign-up for Dan's daily REYNOLDS UNWRAPPED e-mail cartoon for only $12 for a whole year. E-mail Dan at reynoldsunwrapped@gmail.com for details. Dan's website is **www.reynoldsunwrapped.weebly.com**

The Fart Side series and other items are available at:
www.thefunnysidecollection.com

The Funny Side Collection

Joseph Weiss, M.D.

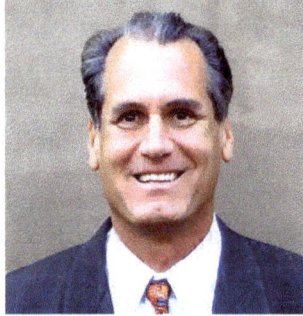

GI Joe is Clinical Professor of Medicine in the Division of Gastroenterology, Department of Medicine, at the University of California, San Diego. He is a Fellow of the American College of Physicians, Fellow of the American Gastroenterological Association, and a Senior Fellow of the American College of Gastroenterology. Dr. Weiss is the author of several dozen books on health, and is an accomplished professional speaker and humorist. His website is: **www.smartaskbooks.com**

"Dr. Joseph Weiss' books provide an informative and entertaining approach to sharing insights about our digestive system and wellbeing." Deepak Chopra, MD

"Joseph Weiss, M.D. has a gift for books that are uniquely informative and entertaining. Jack Canfield Coauthor of the Chicken Soup for the Soul® serie**s**

The Fart Side series and other items are available at:
www.thefunnysidecollection.com

The Fart Side: Life is a Gas!

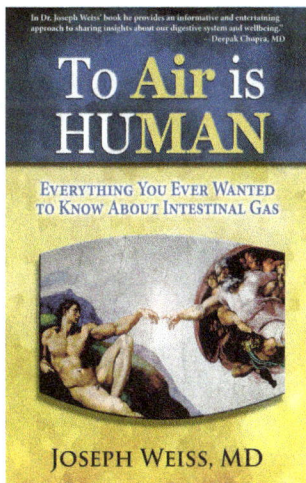

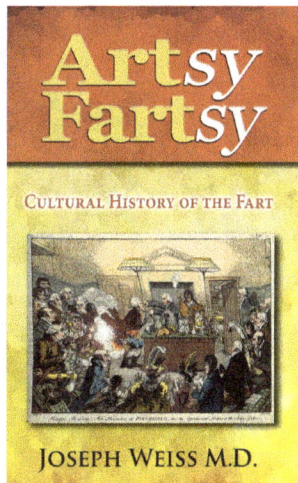

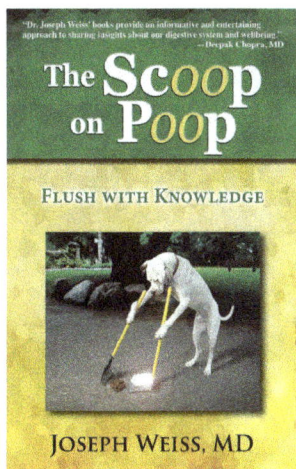

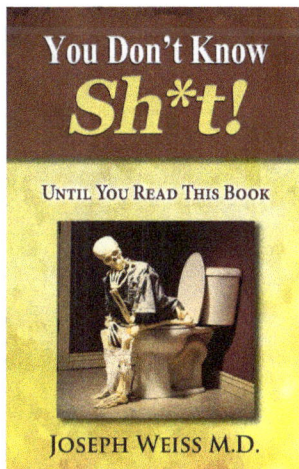

To Air is HUMAN
"In Dr. Joseph Weiss' book he provides an informative and entertaining approach to sharing insights about our digestive system and wellbeing."
— Deepak Chopra, MD
EVERYTHING YOU EVER WANTED TO KNOW ABOUT INTESTINAL GAS
JOSEPH WEISS, MD

Artsy Fartsy
CULTURAL HISTORY OF THE FART
JOSEPH WEISS M.D.

The Scoop on Poop
"Dr. Joseph Weiss' books provide an informative and entertaining approach to sharing insights about our digestive system and wellbeing."
— Deepak Chopra, MD
FLUSH WITH KNOWLEDGE
JOSEPH WEISS, MD

You Don't Know Sh*t!
UNTIL YOU READ THIS BOOK
JOSEPH WEISS M.D.

www.smartaskbooks.com

The Funny Side Collection

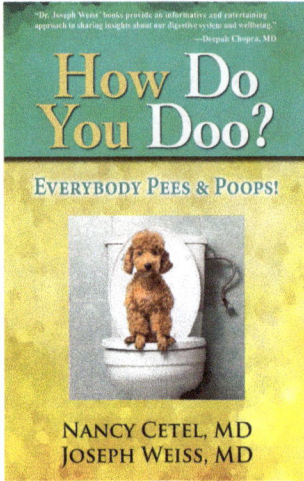

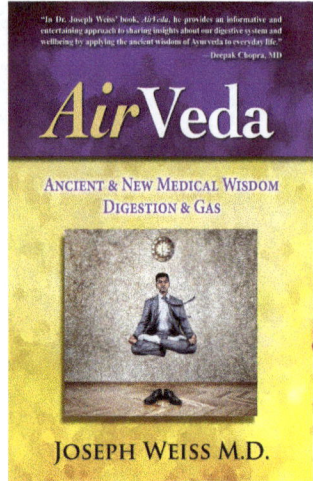

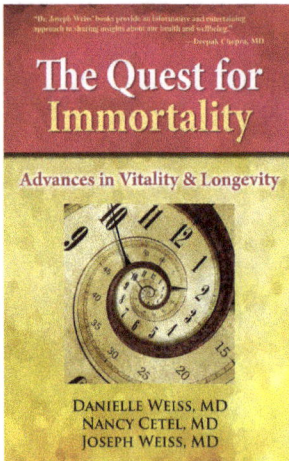

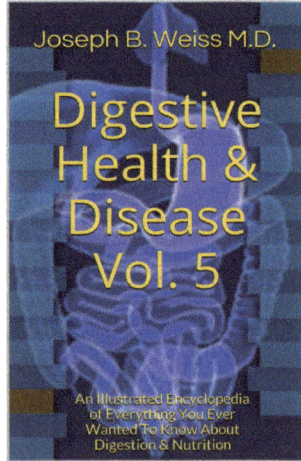

How Do You Doo?

"'Dr. Joseph Weiss' books provide an informative and entertaining approach to sharing insights about our digestive system and wellbeing."
—Deepak Chopra, MD

EVERYBODY PEES & POOPS!

NANCY CETEL, MD
JOSEPH WEISS, MD

Air Veda

"In Dr. Joseph Weiss' book, *AirVeda*, he provides an informative and entertaining approach to sharing insights about our digestive system and wellbeing by applying the ancient wisdom of Ayurveda to everyday life."
—Deepak Chopra, MD

**ANCIENT & NEW MEDICAL WISDOM
DIGESTION & GAS**

JOSEPH WEISS M.D.

The Quest for Immortality

"Dr. Joseph Weiss' books provide an informative and entertaining approach to sharing insights about our health and wellbeing."
—Deepak Chopra, MD

Advances in Vitality & Longevity

DANIELLE WEISS, MD
NANCY CETEL, MD
JOSEPH WEISS, MD

Digestive Health & Disease Vol. 5

Joseph B. Weiss M.D.

An Illustrated Encyclopedia of Everything You Ever Wanted To Know About Digestion & Nutrition

www.smartaskbooks.com

www.ingramcontent.com/pod-product-compliance
Lightning Source LLC
Chambersburg PA
CBHW071242020426
42333CB00015B/1588